"In her beautifully written new book, *Stuck in a Role*, Diana Feldman meticulously offers her formidable method of working with traumatized children through drama and theatre. In discussing her ENACT methodology, Diana lays out its theoretical framework, building upon Bessel Van der Kolk's notion of developmental trauma and many of the key building blocks of drama therapy. She has deeply touched thousands of young lives in her 30 years as a pioneer in drama therapy. In this book, she provides abundant examples to illustrate how and why the ENACT Method is so powerful. This book is a gem and should be read by all who aim to integrate creative methodologies in education, health, medicine, theatre and therapy."

Robert Landy, *PhD, Professor Emeritus, Founding Director, Drama Therapy Program, New York University*

"In Diana Feldman's Introduction in *Stuck in a Role*, she details specific ways that the ENACT practices of this book make a dramatic difference for teachers, teaching artists, administrators, therapists and counselors, and parents. She's exactly right; she's *understating* what a difference this book can make—I know this work, I know what ENACT has accomplished, and I know the difference this book can make for the lives of so many struggling young people. Diana Feldman developed these approaches over decades of masterful practice, and now she thoughtfully and effectively offers these tools to the wider field. We need these tools, and this book delivers. The increases in young people's emotional and psychological stress and trauma are no secret to educators and parents, and it is my fervent hope this book finds its place as a powerful answer to the questions of how to help our most troubled young people. Please study this book carefully and use the solutions it provides."

Eric Booth, *author, global educator, and youth creativity advocate*

"After reading *Stuck in a Role*, we understand how ENACT enables teens to get a second chance in life. As *Stuck in a Role* points out, being a teen comes with a complex set of development behaviors which by adding layers of trauma and emotional neglect only compounds their troubles hoisting up a slew of red flags for the adults who work with them. Teachers and parents often label the disruptive youth and relate to them 'as if' they are that particular behavior or diagnosis. The second chances that Diana Feldman illustrates show us how to get out of the role they are given by others and find their authentic, viable self, which can safely transition into young adulthood.

When we say 'acting out,' we often think of negative behaviors. In reality, youth are acting out their inner conflicts unconsciously trying to undo the damage that has been done to them. By becoming more aware of their feelings in a safe theatrical fashion, students in the ENACT program are able to make better choices in relation to others and themselves. As the inaugural Director of School Mental Health for 15 years in the NYC public schools, I was able to witness firsthand the powerful work of ENACT and the improvement of the students in the program. This book is more than role-play suggestions. Through nuance, connection and compassion, youth become equipped with alternative means in decision making and engaging others in a non-threatening objective manner.

Stuck in a Role reminds us that the body is the first ego the child uses to mediate reality and fantasy. For those students who have experienced trauma, their memories and experiences are contained within—ENACT exercises free up the body so that the emotions come out—a way to verbalize the unspoken. Reading *Stuck in a Role*, I couldn't help thinking of the roles assigned to us, these *assigned identities* and how in our adult life, we need to shake them off seeking that ever present but hard to obtain, true self. We witness students entering her classes in one assigned role and through the art of drama leave with a new, more positive one.

Diana Feldman lays out *Stuck in a Role* in an easy-to-follow structure making complex concepts accessible no matter what your level of expertise so that you too can partake of the tools and interventions for your students, patients, and children alike. By offering the basics of how the brain, emotions, and trauma work as a bundle within the troubled youth, Feldman gives you the keys to unlock the root causes of the trauma and the deprivation the students experience. This will become an indispensable book for years to come.

Schools have to deal with crises and emergencies every day; however, a lot more drama takes place and staff has to discern which is which. *Stuck in a Role* supports teens to experiment with managing their feelings in a safe holding environment allowing them to experience new emotions without getting hit, yelled out or dismissed. By incorporating the ENACT Method, students are able to verbalize their pent-up emotions, name it, and analyze the causes. This newly found awareness allows them to accept the emotion normalizing it as part of the human condition."

Scott Bloom, *Director of Special Projects & Initiatives, New York Psychotherapy and Counseling Center (NYPCC)*

"Finding a way to connect with troubled teens is a complicated task. Diana Feldman has mastered that task, and, in this book, she generously shows us how it can be done. ENACT, the powerful program that Feldman has implemented for 30 years in public schools, is a method using drama therapy that helps students with emotional and psychological pain due to trauma feel a renewed connection to themselves and others, while helping them understand that they are an agent of change in their own lives. Through lively classroom scenes and case vignettes, Feldman illustrates how she helps students understand and have compassion for their behaviors such as aggression, chaos-making, distraction and hopelessness. She helps them realize the underlying meaning underneath their seemingly destructive actions and gives them the sense that they can rewrite their stories and take on new, more positive roles. One can tell from her empathic, attuned writing that Feldman is an adept therapist and talented actor who can really "read the room." Feldman gives plenty of pointers and guidance for the reader who would like to implement the program, or even try out some of the useful activities as a way to help students connect and understand themselves better. If schools implement Feldman's ENACT program in 'behavior disordered' classrooms, our schools would have students who could turn their hardships into healing and make positive contributions to society. I recommend the book to anyone working with children."

Dafna Lender, *LCSW, Certified Trainer and Supervisor/*
Theraplay and DDP, EMDR Therapist

"Consolidating years of knowledge from working with hundreds of thousands of youths, *Stuck in a Role* is a must have resource for any educator or teaching artist looking to use drama to develop students' social emotional skills. The central premise of the book, that students who have experienced trauma are 'stuck in a role,' reminds us all of the power of the arts to help students reimagine the person they are and learn to interact with themselves and the world in ways that are constructive, empowered, and ultimately healing. *Stuck in a Role* draws from extensive psychological research around attachment theory, developmental psychology and neuroscience to present a compelling case that every child can grow their social emotional skills, and that drama is an important avenue for that development. From research, to practice, to individual case studies, this is a book that will sit within arm's reach on my shelf to inform my work."

David Adams, *Chief Executive Officer, Urban Assembly and*
CASEL Board Member

"Diana Feldman's book, *Stuck in a Role*, takes the reader into the minds and emotions of teenagers using the lens of trauma and attachment theories, revealing their complexity and poignancy. Feldman is perhaps the most experienced practitioner of drama therapy in schools in the world, and she brings her expertise and insight to every page. Filled with detailed case examples, lesson plans, theatre games, and step-by-step instructions, this book provides therapists, theatre artists, school counselors, and teachers with the necessary information to develop effective programs for struggling teens. Written in an especially clear and organized style, the book reminds us of the eager, yearning, passionate moments of adolescence, and the wonder in that transition from childhood to adulthood. Diana Feldman's work is a must-read!"

David Read Johnson, *PhD, RDT-BCT,*
Institute for Developmental Transformations

"In *Stuck in a Role: Releasing Trauma in Teens*, Diana J. Feldman presents a groundbreaking approach to healing troubled adolescents. Drawing on 30 years of experience as a drama therapist in New York City schools, Feldman presents the powerful ENACT model, which harnesses the transformative potential of theater to address both individual and collective trauma.

This book illuminates how teens often become trapped in a variety of accommodating and protective roles developed to navigate challenging environments, inadvertently reinforcing negative behaviors. Feldman's innovative method employs play, experimentation, and rehearsal to help young people break free from these confining roles, build crucial relational skills, and find new ways of being. *Stuck in a Role* offers a vital resource for educators, therapists, and anyone seeking to understand and support traumatized teens."

Jack Saul, *PhD, Director, International Trauma Studies*
Program, author of Collective Trauma, Collective Healing

"Theater gives teens a voice; they can say through a role, what they cannot say in real life. It is wonderful that Diana put her successful program ENACT into a form that can allow it to be used more widely to heal teens and to ignite their passion for personal expression going forward."

Tian Dayton, *PhD, TEP, RTR, Creator of Relational Trauma*
Repair (RTR) and author most recently of Treating Adult
Children of Relational Trauma

Stuck in a Role

Stuck in a Role illustrates how adolescents, especially those who have experienced developmental trauma, can become "stuck" in protective roles that can distance them from their authentic selves, and how the ENACT Drama Therapy Method can help them break free from these confining roles.

Using innovative methods of dramatic play, improvisation, and finely honed methods of communication, Feldman shares her unique method of drama therapy, developed over more than 30 years working in the NYC school system, as well as her moving and inspiring case histories.

This book will support all professionals working with children and adolescents, including creative arts educators and therapists, psychotherapists, school counselors, parents, and teachers. It illustrates how to help teens learn crucial coping and relationship skills, moving them toward new and productive ways of being. Through compelling case histories based on Feldman's work with thousands of adolescents labeled hard-to-reach, this book models empathy for youth behavior.

Diana J. Feldman is a Licensed Creative Arts Therapist (LCAT), a Registered Drama Therapist (RDT), and a Board-Certified Trainer (BCT) residing in New York City. She is the creator of the ENACT Drama Therapy Method and has a private practice in New York City.

Stuck in a Role

Releasing Trauma in Teens through the ENACT Drama Therapy Method

Diana J. Feldman

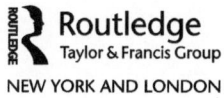
Routledge
Taylor & Francis Group

NEW YORK AND LONDON

Designed cover image: design ©Wendy Boudin/ra2studio/iStock

Editor: Stacey Luftig

First published 2025
by Routledge
605 Third Avenue, New York, NY 10158

and by Routledge
4 Park Square, Milton Park, Abingdon, Oxon, OX14 4RN

Routledge is an imprint of the Taylor & Francis Group, an informa business

Library of Congress Cataloging-in-Publication Data
Names: Feldman, Diana J., author.
Title: Stuck in a role : releasing trauma in teens through the ENACT drama therapy method / Diana J. Feldman.
Description: New York, NY : Routledge, 2025. | Includes bibliographical references and index. |
Identifiers: LCCN 2024052625 (print) | LCCN 2024052626 (ebook) | ISBN
9781032540740 (hbk) | ISBN 9781032540733 (pbk) | ISBN 9781003415022 (ebk)
Subjects: LCSH: Drama--Therapeutic use. | Psychic trauma in children--Treatment. | Psychic trauma in adolescence--Treatment.
Classification: LCC RJ505.P89 F45 2025 (print) | LCC RJ505.P89 (ebook) |
DDC 618.92/8521--dc23/eng/20250314
LC record available at https://lccn.loc.gov/2024052625
LC ebook record available at https://lccn.loc.gov/2024052626

ISBN: 9781032540740 (hbk)
ISBN: 9781032540733 (pbk)
ISBN: 9781003415022 (ebk)

DOI: 10.4324/9781003415022

Typeset in Galliard
by KnowledgeWorks Global Ltd.

I dedicate this book to the thousands of young people ENACT had the opportunity to serve. This work developed through them. Their courage and resilience gave me hope that transformation is possible even under the most challenging circumstances.

Thank you.

Contents

Foreword

Those who work in the fields of expressive arts therapy and creative arts therapies have long known that dramatic enactment is restorative for body and mind. But long before the formal discipline of psychotherapy and arts-based therapies appeared, humans incorporated drama within ceremonies, rituals, and performances as ways of transforming difficulties when confronted by crisis, tragedy, or loss. As a species, we have been turning to the healing factors found in these practices to confront and resolve distress for thousands of years. These actions emerged not only as individual forms of reparation, but also as social engagement, capitalizing on connection with others and community as agents of repair. As a result, drama therapy, psychodrama, and other forms of therapeutic enactment have been acknowledged as effective methods to address and resolve traumatic stress.

And yet, the task of addressing the impact of trauma on young individuals often seems daunting at best. Some of the toughest child client cases I have encountered are those children and teens who have witnessed domestic violence or have directly experienced abuse, neglect, or abandonment. They are survivors who have come face to face with horrors of watching a parent being controlled and abused. This often includes seeing or personally experiencing hitting, shoving, verbal and physical threats, and other forms of assault. Watching one's caregiver be injured leaves young people with at least two dominant narratives. On the one hand, children want to protect their parent from harm and on the other, they simultaneously need to feel protected from violence by the parent. When an altercation between a parent and a partner, or child physical or sexual abuse is reported, there are also other narratives that emerge. They include stories of leaving home, being brought to a community facility like a safe house or shelter, entering foster care, and complicated scenarios involving child protective services, law enforcement, and medical personnel.

When I started to work with children and adolescents who had developmental trauma, I began to notice a sharp contrast in how imagination was expressed compared to individuals without adverse childhood experiences. Some children and teens simply did not know how to interact with toys, art materials, drums, or puppets because they never had these experiences early in life nor guidance from a supportive adult caregiver. Many were too fearful of repercussions or punishment to freely play, pretend, improvise, or make art. I quickly realized that it would be a challenge for these young clients to engage in the very processes that I believed would bring about reparation and a sense of well-being because their ability to imagine was essentially impaired.

Despite these challenges, using drama and pretend play are, in my experience, the most effective ways to work with anyone "stuck" in unproductive trauma stories, as Diana Feldman so expertly and movingly explores in *Stuck in a Role: Releasing Trauma in Teens through the ENACT Drama Therapy Method*. When it comes to dramatic enactment, it is impossible to separate play from drama or acting from play and imagination; they are essentially part of all work with traumatized children and adolescents. They enable individuals to embody various characters, use distancing to pretend, provide opportunities to personify others, and most of all, a chance to imagine new scenarios. They are key approaches that support the transformative work necessary to help young clients make sense and eventually make meaning and transform meaning in their lives. Within the array of creative and expressive arts approaches, drama, enactment, roleplay, and improvisation are the only ones that provide this type of transformative container to literally alter painful and traumatic life narratives.

While children and teens who witness or are subjugated to interpersonal violence have accumulated stories that often require additional support throughout their lives, there are opportunities to help them find islands of relief through imagination and particularly dramatic enactment due to the action-oriented nature of this approach. Simply put, it provides windows for meaning making through the multi-sensory ways not found through verbal counseling or psychotherapy alone.

As a trauma specialist, I believe the kinds of restorative cognitions, emotions, and sensory experiences we want to make "stick" with clients when using art-based approaches are key to eventually helping them imagine new narratives, post-trauma. In other words, if we do not eventually help individuals move away from distress, we leave them with thoughts, feelings, and sensations that will not support new narratives of pleasure, confidence, and hope. This premise is also emphasized in current somatic approaches, which re-sensitize body and mind and develop the capacity for positive emotion through engagement with the body (Malchiodi, 2022). Within the field of expressive arts therapy and creative arts therapies, dramatic enactment in the form of drama therapy uniquely integrates multiple pathways for supporting novel and reparative stories and restoring health and well-being in an action-oriented way.

But as you may wonder—just why is drama therapy such a powerful method? I think there is one obvious answer to this question: It helps individuals find reparation through *performative change*. That is, individuals are engaged in a multilayered, action-oriented process that taps many levels of expression and transformative experiences. Whether improvisation, role play, theatrical reading or actual performance on stage, dramatic enactment generally integrates movement, gesture, sound, voice, playfulness, visual experiences, and storytelling. It provides the opportunity to try out new narratives not only through language, but through the embodiment of a character.

Performative change is central to taking on any dramatic role. But equally important, when experienced as part of a group of actors, there are the added elements of relationships as well as social engagement, attunement, and co-regulation with others. These experiences encourage individuals to take risks through pretend roles and novel identities. When an audience is part of the dynamic, the element of being witnessed is an additional part of the experience both for the individuals playing roles as well as the viewers. What is unique about dramatic enactment in any form is the element of witnessing in the form of audience. In a drama therapy session, the therapist becomes the audience. But in many cases, witnessing takes place in groups, including classrooms, clinics, hospitals, and community centers.

Because dramatic enactment and drama therapy generally occur within groups, the interactions support an important place in work with individuals who have survived trauma. If you have ever worked with groups or in classrooms, you have probably experienced how creative sparks move among participants, igniting new ideas and output. This is particularly helpful for traumatized individuals who may not be able to easily articulate thoughts or feelings; the proximity and interaction experienced through drama naturally stimulate ideas and insights. This is why groups are often more effective for many people whose distress may personal expression, particularly for those who benefit from hearing common experiences and stories of others. It is the key element that makes performative change through drama therapy possible, even for the most traumatized child or adolescent.

In years of work with survivors of interpersonal violence, disasters, or war, I have witnessed individuals who are literally haunted by a theater of sensations in their own bodies, unable to control or articulate how those sensations impact them in multiple and adverse ways. As Feldman describes in this book, drama therapy and the ENACT Drama Therapy Method address and respond to the complex issues that traumatic stress causes and are not easily ameliorated in more cognitive forms of intervention. She skillfully brings together trauma theories with practical guidance on just how drama therapy repairs and transforms young lives.

As a psychotherapist and expressive arts therapist, I understood the field of drama therapy with new clarity through her descriptions and expanded my knowledge of the integrative potentials of dramatic enactment, improvisation, and performance. The principles explained through the ENACT program are ones that all practitioners can integrate into their work not only with children and adolescents, but with people of all ages.

Stuck in a Role sets a new standard for how practitioners, teachers, and even parents and caregivers can envision the treatment of traumatic stress through action-oriented, multi-sensory, and imagination-based methods. It expands our knowledge of creative and expressive methods and just how they can be applied to resolving the mind-body-spirit experience of traumatic stress. More importantly, this book provides readers with a framework for establishing a road map to introducing youth to ways of discovering, creating, and manifesting new narratives that are once resilient, reparative, and restorative.

Cathy A. Malchiodi, PhD
Author, *Trauma and Expressive Arts Therapy:*
Brain, Body, and Imagination in the Healing Process

References

Malchiodi, Cathy A. *Handbook of Expressive Arts Therapy*. New York: Guilford Publications, 2022.

Preface

My intention in writing this book is to offer a new lens for understanding youth behavior as a creative expression of unhealed trauma. I hope that readers will gain a unique insight into youth's creative abilities and view them as talented actors creating roles played out on life's stage as a means of survival, and in doing so, will help them discover their authentic selves.

My journey toward writing this book started when I was a child, with the joy I felt in watching and participating in theater. At about age nine, my grandfather took me to see my first play, *The Prince and the Pauper*. I still remember the excitement in the theater that day when the two lead actors made a surprise entrance from the back of the theater. They walked down the aisles, interacting with various audience members. When he reached me, one of them introduced himself (in character), smiling and shaking my hand before stepping up to the stage. I felt so special! I was hooked, and ready for the magical theatrical experience about to unfold. I didn't know then that this experience would be core to the methods I would develop decades later as a drama therapist.

I also recall the joy of participating in a children's theater group; I loved the spontaneity of performing various roles and the in-the-moment experience of playing theater games. One day, the instructor asked us to call on our imaginations to engage in a creative journey. She guided us through imaginary forests and spaceships to search for lost treasures. On a giant ship in the deep seas, I was enrolled as a pirate with an eye patch searching for lost treasure. Our gang of pirates found the lost treasure chest buried at the bottom of the sea, and we excavated it. We opened the golden box and discovered the shining pearls and diamonds, picking them up and feeling their imaginary textures.

As the session ended, the instructor told us something I would never forget: Deep within ourselves is an invisible treasure chest; we only need to find and open it to reveal our gifts.

The concept of having something unique to discover within ourselves would come up again at a traumatic turning point in my life. I went on to study theater at college. In the middle of the night after graduation day, I was asleep in the back seat of a car packed with friends, returning from a party, when the unthinkable happened: a drunk driver slammed into us, totaling our car.

When I woke up, I was lying on the floor of the car, screaming in pain, broken and twisted. I was unable to move as ambulance workers cut me out of the car. I went from experiencing excruciating pain to suddenly feeling absolutely nothing. My entire body was numb. Terrified, I asked the rescuer if I was paralyzed, and he tried to assure me that I wasn't. But I didn't believe him; I visualized myself paralyzed for the rest of my life.

This concept was unbearable, and I blacked out. But first, I had an epiphany: I was more than the finite boundaries of my body. There was something more profound, something infinite beyond my body. I saw myself singing, tapping into the joy and peace it had always brought me. I realized a creative source existed within me: an unlimited essence. This vision was immediately comforting and gave me the hope needed to cope with the trauma of the very challenging year ahead.

Rushed to the hospital, I was immediately placed on a respirator because my oxygen levels and pulse were quickly fading. I was on the precipice of death when I was suddenly, energetically lifted from my body into a near-death experience that revealed a pure essence beyond the "me" I knew. It was a magnificent, encompassing experience of love. When I returned to my physical self, I felt the heaviness of my body that lay with two shattered legs, a broken arm, and a concussion. I felt hesitant about the choice I made to return to my body, but I knew I had work to do.

I was confined to a body cast for months, during which I felt helpless, frustrated, and frozen.

After being removed from the confining body cast, I slowly learned to walk again, like a child, step by step. My body felt like a block of concrete still stuck in its mold.

My emotions, too, were frozen. I often denied how I felt. I put on a brave face, and often acted the role of a clown as a way to deal with overwhelming feelings. The doctors in the hospital did an excellent job of piecing me back together, but I was far from healed. The traumatic experience caused by the car accident left me with symptoms of post-traumatic stress disorder (PTSD): freeze, panic, and dissociation. I desperately wanted to reconnect with my lost sense of self and regain emotions that were blocked by the trauma I still experienced.

One morning, I felt inspired to pick up my guitar and sing, and when I sang, I was reminded of how free I felt during my epiphany the night of the accident. I intuitively knew that I needed the medicine of the creative arts I had experienced early in my life if I was going to heal. The mask I had created, portraying everything as fine, was not sustainable. I needed to rediscover my authentic self. I knew the creative arts would be my cure.

I worked diligently with dedicated and compassionate healers through movement, music, and other art disciplines. It was a long process, but each embrace of a creative arts approach allowed me another opportunity to heal. The process slowly restored the mental, physical, and spiritual balance I desperately craved. Without knowing it, these compassionate healers were using a powerful approach now appreciated by trauma experts as "bottom-up" healing (a somatic experience integrating the body and the emotions). As my needs felt recognized and my progress was witnessed by my healers, my frozen body armor slowly melted away, as did my exaggerated masks of bravery and humor. My defended emotions were replaced with authentic feelings of sadness and joy.

A year later, I realized my life calling: to develop a creative way to help others work through their trauma and heal by using creative drama to integrate lost parts of themselves. The original inspiration from my childhood theater experiences and my healing journey became the guide to creating the ENACT Drama Therapy Method.

My journey led me to solidify three core concepts. One: Theater is magical. Two: We are more than our minds and physical body; we are a creative, unlimited essence. Three: The arts are a powerful form of medicine that can help us reclaim our authenticity.

The drama therapy approach presented in the following pages offers powerful insights into youth expression and a method of healing for those suffering from unrecognized trauma. I hope that with this perspective and the tools offered in this book, readers will be better equipped to understand and reach out with compassion to the teens in their lives.

In this book, I alternate between he/she and they pronouns to ensure inclusivity and acknowledge the diversity of identities. I aim to create a space where everyone feels seen and represented.

Acknowledgments

I express my deepest gratitude to everyone who contributed to this book. First, I must thank the multitude of teens, parents, teachers, and teaching artists I had the honor to work with for over three decades. Writing the case histories brought back memories I will forever hold dear.

The seed for *Stuck in a Role* was planted over 30 years ago when I consulted with colleagues and friends about creating a non-profit organization to deliver a therapeutic creative drama intervention program to work in schools with young people. My supporters' enduring support and dedication have been a constant source of inspiration for me.

I am incredibly grateful to my teachers and friends who helped me on my healing journey after a life-changing car accident, which led me on a path to fulfill my life's mission. Thank you, Mary Lundy, for teaching me that dance can heal, and Dr. Joyce Parks, who taught me to trust my innate abilities and inner resilience. Special thanks to Dr. Robert Landy, author and Founding Emeritus of the NYU Drama Therapy program. He has been my mentor and friend for over 30 years. I also want to acknowledge Renée Emunah for her drama therapy model, which influenced the framework for this book. I thank my longtime friends for their ongoing support: Wendy Boudin, Fionn Reilly, Jessica Chanin, Jodi Serota, Ellen Abrams, Patti Schaeffer, Priya Sahani, and Lizzie Atlas. I am grateful to my entire family, especially my brilliant sister, Dr. Julie Feldman-Abe, who assisted me with editing suggestions and who has been my cheering squad every step of the way, and my brother Micah Feldman, who was a great support as well. Heartfelt thanks to the talents of Wendy, a graphic artist who designed the book cover, and her detailed work on checking the proofs, and to Fionn, for his beautiful photography.

I am so grateful to my editor, Stacey Luftig, a talented theater lyricist and librettist who endured revision after revision with me, and without whom this book would not have been possible. Thanks to Amy Gottlieb for her invaluable guidance and to Amanda Savage and Sophie Dracott for their ongoing support from Routledge (Taylor & Francis Group). Thank you, Traci Parks, for helping me write the proposal that led to this book. I am so grateful to Arthur McGrath, a gifted therapist who generously contributed his time and expertise in trauma to this book. Special thanks to the readers of my book who gave me invaluable feedback. Thank you, Mimi Savage and Scott Bloom, and a heartfelt thanks to my longtime advisor and friend, Eric Booth, an avid champion in arts education. Thank you, David Adams, for your contributions to social-emotional learning. Thank you, Dr. Jack Saul, for your work in collective trauma. Thank you, David Read Johnson, for your wise input and support. I am grateful to Tian Dayton and Dafna Lender for their guidance and support. Finally, I want to thank all the talented ENACT actor-teachers and drama therapists, many of whom were with me for over a decade. Special recognition goes to Emilie Ward, Emily Weiner, and Miles Grose for your longtime commitment and contribution to the ENACT Method. Thank you, Betty Graham and Cristina Hernandez, for your resilience and humor when we needed it most. Special thanks to Andrea Aranguren and Alicia Thompson for your talents and commitment.

I thank Jeffrey Davis, a talented author and thought leader. He deserves credit for his poetic writing contributions to the case histories. Thank you, Cathy Malchiodi, founder of the Expressive Arts Therapist Institute, for writing the forward to this book.

I am grateful to all the teachers, administrators, and advisors from the New York City Department of Education who supported ENACT all these years. ENACT would not have been possible without generous funding from the New York City Council and the Ford Foundation. Mason Granger from the Hearst Foundation and Danielle Pulliam from the Pinkerton Foundation lent generous support, encouragement, and belief in the ENACT program. Thank you!

About the Author

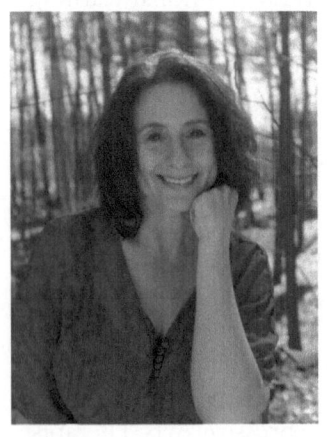

Diana Jeanne Feldman is a Licensed Creative Arts Therapist (LCAT), a Registered Drama Therapist (RDT), and a Board-Certified Trainer (BCT) residing in New York City. She founded ENACT Inc. and created the ENACT Method, which served over 250,000 students, parents, and teachers in New York City schools for over 30 years. She trains teachers, therapists, teaching artists, and parents nationwide and internationally. Ms. Feldman has won numerous awards, including a five-year Ford Foundation Grant, to demonstrate the efficacy of her evidence-based method. Ms. Feldman has spoken at mental health and education conferences nationwide and abroad, authored multiple articles in drama therapy journals, and contributed chapters in drama therapy books and creative arts therapy books. Ms. Feldman is passionate about helping children and does volunteer work with children and families in rural areas of India. She resides in New York City and has a private practice working with children, teens, and families.

Introduction

It is our first day with a new group of students. My partner Charles and I need to grab their attention and engage them right away if we're to succeed. We don't yet have a particular student to focus on, as we usually do, but we know that our teacher/student scene usually resonates with almost all the students.

I enter first, playing the role of the teacher. The classroom is in chaos. Only a few students are sitting at their desks. Most are roaming the room, talking, laughing, and throwing paper airplanes. They barely notice me.

Charles, playing the role of Troy, The Class Clown, comes galloping in, headphones on, dancing to the music. I portray Mrs. Jones, the agitated teacher, and yell over the kids' voices.

"You are late again, Troy!" I bark at him.

"What did you say?" he shouts.

"Take off your headphones," I say.

"I can't hear you," he yells, "I have my headphones on."

"Take them off!" I yell louder as he removes them.

"Ouch, you are hurting my ears and yelling too loud."

The kids in the audience are watching, and some don't get the joke and need clarification. Others laugh. We have caught their attention!

I ask the students, "Do you know who we are?" They have no idea because no one told them we were coming. We explain that we are actors and were asked to work with them in their classroom. A student approaches me, laughing with a comical voice. He says, "Because we are the bad kids, right?"

"Well," I respond, "we're interested in working with you because I have been told you are good actors, right?"

"I guess," he says. "I can act like a student," he says, laughing.

"So should we continue?" I ask.

"I guess," he says again.

DOI: 10.4324/9781003415022-1

I address the class. "We need quiet to finish the scene. Is that OK? Maybe you could help us move the chairs into a semicircle and create a theater space. What do you think?" The kids look at each other, and some move the chairs. Peter, a tall, lanky boy, is busy fidgeting at his desk and doesn't hear me. I decide to let him stay where he is.

"We need a director to say 'Quiet on the set,' and only when it is quiet, say 'Action!' OK?"

We take our places in front of the chalkboard, poised to begin. A student raises his hand. "I'll be the director," he says. "Quiet on the set... Action!" He nods, and we begin.

We start the scene from the top. Troy roams around the room, talking and laughing with one classmate after another. "Did you watch that show last night?" Troy says loudly to a classmate. "Wasn't it corny?" Troy laughs, moves on to another classmate, and even sits in their lap, cracking jokes and purposely undermining the teacher's authority. As the teacher, I become increasingly annoyed. "Don't pay attention to him," I tell the class. "He just wants attention; ignore him." Knowing this would resonate with them, Troy moves strategically around the room, shoring up the attention he needs from his peers. Moving like a flamenco dancer, he lands in Peter's lap. Peter is laughing. Troy returns to the front of the class and stands next to me.

"Troy," I say, "did you do your homework?"

"I don't have it," he says.

"Where is it?" I ask.

"It's at home. Get it? It's homework, so it is at home!"

He laughs. He looks at his peers for validation as they laugh with him.

"That's not funny," I say. "You think you are funny, but you are not!"

Now I'm yelling. I move closer to him, and he backs away. I move closer again and put my hand on his shoulder. "Please sit down now!"

This is the trigger that pushes Troy to become emotionally explosive. "Get your hands off me," he says, holding up his fist as if he will hit me. "Who do you think you are, my mother?"

The scene stops at this conflict point. We face the audience in a frozen position.

"Inside!" I call out.

The room is silent. The students are now transfixed. Even Peter raises his head from the desk and watches.

Troy speaks directly to the audience. In an inner monologue, he expresses his unspoken turmoil and core feeling of hopelessness.

She better never touch me again, or I'll hurt her! Who does she think she is, my mother? I don't have my homework. I have no time to do it. My dad is in jail, and my mom works all night, so I have to watch my little brother. I'm late for school? I live an hour and a half away and have to take my little brother to school first. Sometimes, I don't even want to get out of bed in the mornings cause I'm all nervous, just thinking and thinking about everything. Who cares about school anyway? I'm just gonna fail. This teacher better stop picking on me; I'm telling you, I'll mess her up!!

End scene. We begin the inquiry phase: "Does this look familiar? Is it realistic?"

The scenario above illustrates one of the many ways that my drama therapy organization, ENACT, would engage a new group of students, and is part of a case history that you will read in its entirety in Chapter 10. I founded ENACT (Educational Network of Artists in Creative Theater) in the late 1980s. Back then, we were a small, New York City-based arts and education program, a team of six actors, eager to use our skills in improvisational theater to work with kids in school classrooms.

Over the next 30 years, ENACT grew into a nonprofit organization with over 60 teaching artists (some of whom grew up in the same neighborhoods as our students), drama therapists, and social workers working in hundreds of classrooms across New York City's five boroughs.

ENACT served over 250,000 students, many of whom were labeled as "acting out." We soon realized these behaviors were a sign of something far deeper and came to understand that in many—if not most—cases, we were dealing with symptoms of unrecognized trauma. As our methods for addressing these symptoms evolved, ENACT's success in reaching these students continued to grow, and ENACT was soon called a "program of choice" by the New York City Department of Education. We were called into classrooms to work with students with behavior problems, some of whom were deemed "unreachable" and were often sent to school hospital programs and suspension centers. As we grew, much of our work took place in alternative schools and other specialized youth centers.

These students were not unreachable. They were *"stuck in a role."* Through the ENACT Drama Therapy Method, we were able to help many of them release their symptoms of trauma and help them return to their authentic selves.

Welcome to *Stuck in a Role*, **a book about dramatic youth transformation.** You may be a teacher, a therapist, a program administrator, or a group leader in a nonclinical setting. You may be a parent or caregiver of a foster child, an adopted child, or a child that is born to you. And you are almost certainly a caring, brave adult who wants to help youth. You see them acting out through challenging behaviors and are concerned that they are suffering. But what if they don't want your help? What if they oppose or reject your attempts? Don't lose hope!

Stuck in a Role will offer you insights and techniques to work directly with teens by viewing them through a fresh lens. You will appreciate them as actors playing roles in their attempts to communicate and manage difficult emotions and symptoms of trauma. By learning new techniques, you can help guide the young people in your life toward insights that can help free them from defensive behaviors that don't serve them. At the same time, you can help them get in touch with and heal the vulnerable parts they are protecting and provide them with valuable coping skills. In essence, you can assist them in becoming self-aware as they build self-esteem, communicate more effectively, and relinquish defensive patterns that keep them "stuck in a role."

The methods described in *Stuck in a Role* have been formally vetted. In 2008, ENACT was awarded a five-year research grant from the Ford Foundation to observe our methods. A team of researchers from the Center for Arts Education Research at Teachers College at Columbia University conducted an evidence-based study that concluded, "Students became more aware of their feelings and behavior and were often able to express or dramatize their feelings in an atmosphere of trust that helped them find solutions to challenging personal situations." These findings were peer-reviewed and presented at the American Evaluation Association in 2011.

Additionally, *85% of participating teachers reported that ENACT improved their classroom environment, and 87% reported that it improved the school climate.* What was most important to us was that the evidence concluded that "ENACT was successful at engaging students by building an atmosphere of trust and paying attention to their needs."

If you are a teacher, this book will help you:

- View behavior through the lens of trauma.
- Learn about trauma symptoms and emotional regulation.
- Understand resistance and learn tools to address it.
- Create a classroom environment built around engagement, trust, and safety.
- Learn user-friendly theater games for all ages and abilities.
- Understand how youth compensate for feeling difficult emotions by developing false selves or roles.

Some of the behaviors that teachers encounter are typical teen responses to classroom situations. But others may be signs of unrecognized trauma. The adolescents who explode when a teacher approaches them may have been emotionally triggered by a memory of something that happened to them months or years before. The student staring out the window may have been bored but could also have been experiencing symptoms of dissociation (a response to stress or exhaustion from trauma). Some students seem entirely out of control. They have dysregulated behavior (difficulty controlling emotions). Symptoms of trauma may look simply like bad behavior. But they are so much more. Students who exhibit these symptoms have nervous systems that are on fire and cannot self-regulate. But you can help these teens to heal and transform.

If you are a teaching artist, **this book will help you:**

• Learn to understand resistance and use time-tested principles to move through it so that you can engage students to fully participate in your program.
• Learn how to create a safe, protective, creative space that supports learning.
• Learn to understand trauma so you can better understand your students' behaviors.
• Implement theater-game activities to engage students immediately and be equipped with sample user-friendly theater techniques that are adjustable for your art form.
• Learn how the arts help to heal through what trauma experts call a bottom-up approach (body-mind healing) and how these skills can help students regulate their nervous systems so they can become engaged in an interactive learning process. You are likely already doing this.

Working as a teaching artist can be very fulfilling; you get to share your craft with enthusiastic young people, and you may possibly be changing lives. But other times, especially when working with students with behavior challenges, the experience of resistance can be overwhelming. Self-doubt, anger, and even feelings of hopelessness can kick in. It's not your fault; you may be the perfect person to help them. You are an unsung hero who can make significant changes in their lives. You can do this!

If you are a program administrator, **this book will help you:**

• Discover a method founded in therapeutic concepts and applied to interactive theater-based activities.

- Understand how trauma may be affecting your staff.
- Locate a program or assemble a team of skilled instructors, such as actors and therapists, to deliver the ENACT Method of drama therapy.
- Locate a trainer to teach your staff interactive ENACT activities like developmental theater games and trauma-based role-play.
- Help your staff learn up-to-date principles in trauma, which they can immediately apply to their own work.

The job of a program administrator can be daunting. You are trying to provide crucial services to many individuals of all ages and abilities and all with different needs. Children, teachers, patients, and clients count on you to provide them with the services they require. You are a juggler, a matchmaker, a fundraiser, and a magician. You really want to help, but sometimes, your job feels overwhelming as you try to meet the needs of so many people. But you do it because you care. And isn't it fulfilling when you know you have provided meaningful services to those who otherwise may never have had the chance to participate in programs like these?

If you are a therapist, this book will help you:

- Read and address youth behavior through role presentation.
- Learn embodied (bottom-up approaches) theater games to address emotional regulation.
- Learn role-play techniques such as inner monologues to heighten self-awareness.
- Learn indirect scene techniques to address resistance.
- Understand the concept of using emotional distance to create a personal connection.
- Help teens to safely relinquish their long-held defenses and reclaim their authenticity.

As you know, clients who are oppositional, shut down, bored, and apathetic are showing you their survival mechanisms and their unique and creative style of self-protection. An innovative, indirect approach employing a discipline outside of your field may be just the medicine they need.

If you are a parent, this book will help you:

- Understand the signs and symptoms of a dysregulated nervous system.
- Co-regulate by learning techniques to regulate your own nervous system.

- Learn to address your child's underlying needs to transform behavior.
- Learn why kids create roles and how to avoid getting caught up in their drama.
- Understand how behavior can be a misguided approach to coping with difficult emotions.
- Improve your relationship with your child by learning the valuable concept of attunement and co-regulation to help them feel seen, heard, and understood.

It can be challenging to be a parent of a developing teen. It's normal for them to be up and down at this time as they transition from childhood to adulthood. Still, if they are experiencing what appears to be extreme symptoms of anxiety and depression, they may need some extra help, and there is no one more committed to their well-being than you.

Whatever involvement you have in the life of teenagers, *Stuck in a Role* can help you learn strategies for reaching them. Part 1 of this book will give you an overview of trauma, symptoms, and strategies, essential for a deeper understanding of the behavior exhibited by so many teens labeled "unreachable." Part 2 provides a step-by-step guide to the ENACT Method, useful for those who want to set up a program in their school or other setting, as well as a shortened version of the same principles that can be used by anyone. The book will end with user-friendly theater games and some lesson plans you can use immediately.

And now... **Quiet on the set. Action!**

Part 1

Foundations for Understanding Teens with Trauma

Chapter 1

Developmental Trauma and Attachment Theory

Aisha collapsed and was sent to the hospital when the gym teacher told her to stop bothering her. Each day, Aisha showed up early in her teacher's office and refused to leave after class. Before that, Aisha had pursued the school principal for months, trying desperately to get her attention and telling her schoolmates that the principal was her loving aunt. Aisha desperately wanted a connection with an adult but didn't know how to get it. She alienated them with her obsessively needy behavior. When all her attempts to connect failed, she gave out and fainted. Aisha was needy for a reason. Her mother had died when she was an infant, and she was shuffled from one foster family to another, never having a place to call home. Motherless, she never had an opportunity for early attachment and sought to fill the void of the love she had never experienced.

*

"Don't look at me, or I'll kill you!" said Jason. He was talking to Lisa, his classmate, in a hospital school program for students who could not function well in a public high school. Lisa would keep her head low and barely look up, afraid of Jason's reaction, but he continued to repeat the same daily threat. It was hard not to notice that Jason's face was covered with throbbing pimples, causing him to feel self-conscious. Jason was teased and bullied regularly by his peers, and his home life was unstable. Dad was in prison, and mom worked two jobs. His tough-guy attitude was designed to protect him, but it only caused further isolation.

*

James was called into the principal's office almost daily because of his attention-seeking, clown-like behavior, which interfered with

DOI: 10.4324/9781003415022-3

the teacher's ability to instruct. He knew his peers enjoyed his boisterous, over-the-top behavior, so he kept it up, gaining more positive feedback through their laughter and sense of approval. His teacher attempted to rein him in, but she was repeatedly unsuccessful. Unable to manage her frustration, she would relegate him to the principal's office. James struggled with depression and had a difficult home life.

———————

The students in the cases above shared a common denominator: the fundamental need to feel safe, seen, and protected—the yearning for emotional connection. Growing up in stressful homes, these adolescents lacked the early bonds of attachment that would give them a secure foundation for their growth and development. As therapist, researcher, and noted author Bessel van der Kolk puts it, "Children whose parents are reliable sources of comfort and strength have a lifetime advantage–a kind of buffer against the worst that fate can hand them."[1] Lacking trust, they were hyper-alert and easily activated by a look or a word, sending them into a tailspin of reactivity. They were acting out their pain and were often labeled as "defiant," "oppositional," or having "conduct disorder."

This was the case with most of the teens I worked with over my 30-plus years as a drama therapist in New York City public schools. These teens lived in urban neighborhoods with high rates of poverty and crime. Most came from unstable homes or living conditions, and many had experienced neglect and abuse. But they were also resourceful and resilient. They developed adaptive behavior in response to their stressful environments and strong defenses to shield them from the inner turmoil they were experiencing. Some created false selves or roles to compensate for their negative self-concepts and to fit into peer groups that often served as their only support systems.

When I first created the ENACT method, I wasn't aware of **attachment theory** or the detrimental effects of **developmental trauma**, two foundational concepts that I will explain later in this chapter. When I did come to understand these concepts, they helped deepen my compassion for the behavior I saw in the classrooms where I worked. I have come to realize that it is not unusual for anyone to be touched (at least on some level) by the effects of developmental trauma, even if they grew up in more stable homes and environments.

Understanding developmental trauma and attachment theory can help us make sense of the probable origins of youth's **dysregulated behavior** (trouble controlling emotions), allowing for new possibilities to help them regulate their emotions and learn the skills needed to transform their behavior. I will refer to these concepts throughout this book because they are foundational to teens who have experienced trauma. You will learn that reactive behavior can be a response to unrecognized emotions misunderstood by well-meaning adults who have labeled them as challenging, oppositional, or unreachable. You may even gain insights and develop compassion for your own childhood.

But before we can delve into these core concepts, let's look at the period of adolescence.

Adolescence

Adolescence is an intense time of physical, emotional, and cognitive development. Hormones are changing, and increasing stress levels can make it difficult for young people to control their emotions and moods. Some have called adolescence the "crazy-making stage." One minute, they are laughing and seemingly having fun; the next, they are angry and reactive for no apparent reason. Teens compare themselves with others as they try on new roles and let others go. They are developing their self-concepts.

During adolescence, the brain gradually transforms from that of a child to that of an adult. The brain is only considered fully developed at age 25. Girls generally begin adolescence sooner than males, creating further imbalance and tensions. This is partly why boys are often considered "immature"—they are less mature developmentally than girls of the same age tend to be.

Parents sometimes find their teenagers elusive and hard to read. Many teenagers can't or won't explain how they feel because they may not know and are figuring things out, or they have blocked their feelings to maintain control—keeping thoughts and feelings to themselves. Many teens have strong emotional defenses. They are learning what is safe or unsafe to express and share with others. In adolescence, many behaviors are designed to get attention because they perceive that others are observing them. Other times, behaviors are designed to avoid attention whenever possible. This is because they are often observing themselves.

Many teens want to experience new sensations, and they may take risks that may not be in their best interests. Peer groups become increasingly important to them, and peers can pressure them to try out potentially harmful activities like experimenting with drugs or alcohol and engaging in crime, or to join gangs.

Teens often turn to their peers for support in this state between childhood and adulthood. Peer groups offer friendship and acceptance, which is especially important to youth from unstable homes. As adolescents are individuating from their family systems, peers can provide a critical sense of security and belonging. Teens will work hard to fit in, sometimes denying their own thoughts and feelings.

Teens who have low self-esteem and a negative self-image may develop a role to compensate for parts of themselves that they believe are inadequate.

They may experiment with different kinds of false selves/roles like the ones you will read about in this book, such as the attention-seeking Clown, The Bully who feels powerless, or The Victim, who feels prone to being hurt. (I further explain the use of roles in Chapter 4.)

Yet, despite their efforts for acceptance, teens may experience stress from their peers in forms such as peer pressure, hurtful gossip, or bullying, which can be devastating to their sense of self-worth. As a result of negative peer reactions, they may adjust their self-presentation by dressing a certain way and portraying an attitude, posture, and gestures they deem will be more acceptable. They may rely on a false self to protect their vulnerable self from hurt. In their quest for self-acceptance and acceptance from peers and others, they push aside authentic parts of themselves and replace them with behaviors that can ultimately become habitual, causing them to get **"stuck in a role."** Put another way, their new behavior can cause them to lose an essential connection with themselves.

To further understand adolescents' behavior, it is essential to understand their early childhood experiences. This is where the often-missed concept of developmental trauma comes in.

Developmental Trauma

Bessel van der Kolk introduced a groundbreaking diagnosis called developmental trauma in his book *The Body Keeps the Score*. He describes the long-lasting impact of chronic early trauma and its wide-ranging consequences on physical and emotional development. He explains that developmental trauma speaks to the horrific negative impacts of neglect, lack of empathy, abuse, abandonment, and other injustices from a primary caregiver. The brain's development, emotion regulation, behavioral control, cognition, self-concept, and more are all affected by developmental trauma.[2]

If developmental trauma begins early, when the child's brain is developing and their neural networks are forming, it can cause extensive biological problems, leading to difficulty with cognitive development, self-regulation, and social interactions. In later years, youth can become easily triggered and feel out of control. To cope with intense unregulated emotions, teens try to manage their symptoms in various ways, usually through reactive behavior, becoming dissociated, hyper-alert, or just feeling numb. Some teens without better coping skills may attempt to self-soothe by using drugs, cutting themselves, or engaging in other forms of self-harm.

Parents of children suffering from developmental trauma may, sadly, be suffering themselves and are unable to help their children develop in a healthy way. They may be struggling with substance abuse, unemployment, or other causes of intense stress. In addition, their own unhealed trauma may have left them unable to properly attach to their children or respond to their children's needs, and the cycle continues.

The effects of developmental trauma on youth can be seen in various social contexts such as classrooms, playgrounds, youth centers, hospitals, foster care centers, and other youth settings. This trauma is exhibited not just by the kids who "act out" but also by those who "act in" because trauma often leads to social isolation.

While developmental trauma is not always the culprit, you may have observed this phenomenon in people without knowing it. Maybe a woman snaps at you while she packs up your groceries at the supermarket, or maybe you've observed a child sitting by themselves on a park bench, head down and looking sad, while nearby a group of other kids happily chatter, or maybe you see an adolescent in the street violently lashing out at their girlfriend. This may stem from physical or emotional stress, but it might also be developmental trauma.

Learning about developmental trauma provides a framework to help understand what leads to youth's extreme resistance and reactive behavior.

If you notice an adolescent becoming easily triggered by an unconscious facial expression from you or from a peer or if they are highly resistant to participating in activities that you are conducting, it is a clue that they may be suffering from developmental trauma and negative attachment experiences. Try not to take the behavior personally. By understanding that they are trying to find ways to manage their painful emotions, you can help them learn other, more positive ways to cope with their complicated feelings and new ways to help them feel safe and connected.

Understanding the damaging effects of developmental trauma can help us avoid mislabeling or taking punitive actions against youth exhibiting symptoms used for their emotional survival. We can develop deep empathy and, ultimately, find a more effective treatment for them.

The Adverse Childhood Experiences (ACE) Study

An important study on early childhood experiences illuminates this development period.[3] The Adverse Childhood Experiences (ACE) Study was a groundbreaking analysis of the effects of childhood trauma. It was conducted by Kaiser Permanente and the Centers for Disease Control and Prevention (CDC) from 1995 through 1997 to determine the link between adverse childhood experiences and adult health. It is the most thorough study of its kind and included 17,000 participants.[4] It demonstrates that childhood trauma affects individuals throughout their entire lifespan. Based on a scoring system of questions ranging from issues of neglect to the loss of a parent or family mental illness, the results lead us to the critical understanding that almost no one is untouched by trauma.

The ACE Study also demonstrates that the more adversity we are exposed to as children, the greater the risk we have for addictions, mental health issues, and myriad other medical problems later in life. Adversity factors fall under three categories: abuse, neglect, and family dysfunction.[5]

A more recent survey discovered that at least 52 percent of participating adolescents recognized that they were facing or had faced at least one category of childhood adversity.[6] The study concluded that childhood trauma has a direct correlation to mental and physical health. Based on the results of this study, it is likely that most of us fall somewhere on the ACE scale.

Not just the relevant events in someone's life cause the trauma. The after-effects count as well. The pain of feeling unseen and unheard by a primary caregiver can cause emotional damage that can live within the body until it is, hopefully, addressed. Long-term effects of neglect and abuse affect every cell in the body and affect the nervous system and emotions long after the abuse occurs.

Learning about early childhood trauma can start us on a path to understanding and transforming emotional injury in ourselves and others. Practitioners can search for physical and mental health symptoms that lead to their root cause to help heal wounded parts that may be ignored or denied and help restore integrity and emotional integration.

This information can significantly help practitioners who work with children and adolescents, helping them change initial assumptions and understand their clients' behaviors in new ways.

Practitioners may benefit substantially from becoming familiar with the ACE Study and taking it themselves. The outcomes may come as a surprise or comfort, but they can provide us with an understanding of some of our deepest emotional challenges.

Attachment

Developmental trauma can cause long-term emotional damage, and a problem with early **attachment** is a critical factor in developmental trauma. Early parent-child bonds deeply impact our interpersonal relationships and emotional and social development.

The central tenet of **attachment theory** is that relationships we form with others begin with our first connection with our primary caregivers. We are born as fragile, dependent beings who can only survive with the care of another. A biological connection exists between the caregiver and the infant to serve the physical and emotional needs required for the child to grow and develop. This bond between parent and child is the child's introduction to relationships, and it will impact their relationships throughout their lives. If a parent is responsive to a child's needs through touch and sound, soothing them when they cry, rocking them in their arms, or imitating their natural sounds, the child will feel loved. The child will internalize feelings of safety. Sadly, if the caregivers abuse or neglect the child, the child's sense of safety and trust becomes damaged. The child may have difficulty trusting others and regulating their emotions throughout their lifetime.

No parent is perfect; parents should not feel bad about their mistakes. There will be attachment ruptures from time to time, but the good news is that these mistakes can be repaired. When attachment ruptures are ongoing and they do not get corrected, they can harm or cause harm to a child's emotional development.

In the 1980s, attachment research began to focus on the mal-treatment of children.[7] In 1986, Mary Main and Judith Solomon introduced the concepts of insecure attachment and disorganized attachment, which apply to traumatized children.[8] The theory explains some children's aggressive and avoidant behavior as caused by a lack of proper attachment. This critical finding is important for adults who work with youth, as it can explain the reasons for certain behaviors in children, reduce the need for labeling, provide critical insight, and promote empathy.

Attachment theory explains how a developing child with a positive attachment can handle life's challenges better than those who do not have a positive attachment with a primary caregiver.

Positive attachment provides children with a foundation and a compass for feeling safe and protected. Without it, they are often left without an anchor and with a deep yearning to feel loved and connected. Children who grew up in homes with neglect and abuse suffer terribly from the effects of negative attachment and tend to have an unfulfilled yearning for that primitive connection that can haunt them for the rest of their lives.

Understanding attachment theory can help those of us who work with children to have empathy for how youth relate to others and themselves. Young people may have challenging relationships, especially with adults, if they were wounded by their early relationships with their caregivers. Because of the lack of a strong attachment bond with caregivers, they have a hard time regulating their feelings and managing their moods, leading to difficulties in school and other social environments. Youth may also have trouble being reliable and find themselves simultaneously wanting to stay and to run. Neither option feels safe. They will act out their adverse attachment history through extreme resistance and challenging behavior. These youth are often labeled as having oppositional defiant disorder. Of course, a label such as this one does not explain the cause and can have the effect of writing off behavior as unfixable.

Children who grow up without a caregiver of any kind can experience feelings of helplessness and desperation. This was the case for Aisha, who was introduced at the start of this chapter. She was a young student who lost her mother as an infant and was so desperate for connection that when her efforts for connection with her teachers failed, she had a panic attack and fainted. Her abandonment anxiety was too much for her to bear.

Those who work with children in foster care agencies understand that children who are taken from their homes and placed in these agencies, particularly government programs, will feel an additional loss of connection. Their difficult behavior reflects that attachment wound, and while designed to protect themselves from further injury, their challenging and reactive behavior often causes them to be moved from one home to another.

It may feel difficult to form a connection with a child injured by attachment trauma, but a consistent, caring adult can make an enormous difference.

Foster families can benefit greatly by understanding the concept of attachment because they will realize that their attempts at connection with a foster child may be challenging and sometimes feel impossible. Still, with proper knowledge and understanding, they will learn not to take difficult behavior personally or give up too soon on a relationship that can be saved by a consistent and caring adult.

The effects of unhealed attachment wounds can also be cumulative. Attachment wounds are often passed down from one generation to another. Sadly, this continues a legacy of neglect. The good news is that healing is possible. Positive relationships with caring adults can set up the path. According to Daniel Siegel's book *Mindsight*, "wonderful things happen when people feel felt, when they sense their minds are held within another's mind."[9] Corrective experiences include providing a safe, nurturing environment where a young person can be authentically seen and heard and being responsive to their needs.

It is important to understand that teens who suffer from developmental trauma and early attachment ruptures may live in a state of chronic anxiety, defensiveness, and/or hypervigilance to shield themselves against their own painful, traumatic emotions. In service of their emotional survival, they repress their complex emotions. They communicate and act out their needs through extreme behaviors that challenge authority and oppose adults, which often has the tragic effect of pushing away those who genuinely want to help them.

I hope you will think about the youth you work with or live with and entertain the idea that their dysregulated behavior and trouble relating to adults can be viewed as a map tracing their history. Armed with these new understandings, there are significant ways you can help them, which are introduced in Part 2 of this book. Based on these concepts, you can create your zones of safety and positive attachment experiences that will impact their lives in simple and profound ways. But before such transformations can be fostered, insight is needed into how teens' negative behaviors are triggered and how to better handle these situations.

Notes

1 van der Kolk, *The Body Keeps the Score*, 112.
2 van der Kolk, *The Body Keeps the Score*.
3 Felitti, *Am J Prev Med*. 1998;14(4):245–258.
4 Malchiodi, *Trauma and Expressive Arts Therapy*, 42.
5 Centers for Disease Control and Prevention, Violence Control, About the CDC-Kaiser ACE Study, https://www.cdc.gov/violenceprevention/aces/about.html
6 Katembu, Zahedi, Sommer. *Front Public Health*. 2023;11:1001132. https://doi.org/10.3389/fpubh.2023.1001132
7 Crittenden, *J Child Psychol Psych*. 1985;26(1);85–96; Egeland and Sroufe, *Child Dev*. 1981;52(1):44–52; Schneider-Rosen, *Mon Soc Res Child Dev*. 1985;50(1):194–210.
8 Main and Solomon. Discovery of a new, insecure-disorganized/disoriented attachment pattern. In: Yogman, Brazelton (eds), *Affective Development in Infancy*.
9 Siegel, *Mindsight*, 189.

Chapter 2

Understanding Reactive Behavior in Teens

"What's your name?" I asked a girl among a group of students with "behavioral problems," most of whom had strolled in late to our ENACT workshop.

"I don't know."

"I don't know. I like that name—should I call you that?"

"Yes, that's my name," the girl responded and laughed as if she were mocking me.

I wondered what factors in her story might make this young woman so cautious. I also realized I had not even told anyone my name. I introduced myself.

I worked this day with a group of non-stop chattering, giggling, sarcastic girls. I was assigned to work with their "behavioral challenges" through our interactive drama program. How engaged they were or were not during the initial drama exercises was next to impossible to assess, as barely a genuine comment or gesture slipped from behind their way-cool and sarcastic roles. Natural performers, I thought. It would take work to break through their resistance and develop trust. We needed to prove ourselves to them.

Does this sound familiar? Sometimes, teenagers act like they don't like you and won't connect with you, no matter how hard you try. Michelle did not trust me. She did not trust or like any adult. She inhabited a role I call The Defiant One, refusing to connect and pushing back in countless ways with every adult she encountered. You can read the rest of Michelle's case history at the end of this chapter.

Behavior like Michelle's is very common with teens who have had negative attachment experiences with their early caregivers. Lack of trust

DOI: 10.4324/9781003415022-4

is demonstrated in many ways. Some teens may accuse you of embarrassing or insulting them, and you may have no idea what you did to upset them. So you ask them directly, and they freeze you out. They may ignore and resist every effort you make to get the class to calm down and focus; the more you try, the more the behavior worsens. Then there are those students on the other end of the spectrum. They are excessively clingy, and as much as you want to reciprocate, you feel overwhelmed and unsure of how to respond.

I can assure you that if you have experienced this, you are not alone. I hear these complaints from teachers around the country working with youth in diverse schools, and I have certainly encountered this behavior myself.

After many years of working with teachers struggling with these issues, I came to understand the symptoms of developmental trauma, and the lightbulb went off! The students with extreme reactive behavior were exhibiting symptoms of developmental trauma!

If you work with teens in any capacity, it's essential to understand why they become so easily activated and emotionally dysregulated so that the next time it happens—and it will—you will recognize that their behavior kicks in whenever they perceive they are unsafe in their environment.

For teens who have experienced trauma, this radar system is a result of their complex history. They respond to unrecognized and unresolved internal emotional struggles and cues that began in early childhood. This knowledge alone can help you find new ways to reach them.

Understanding additional concepts can be helpful as well. First, it's important to recognize that the behavior exhibited by teens is not just psychological but physiological. This chapter will cover the concept of **neuroception**, which occurs as an unconscious scanning mechanism to help youth monitor levels of safety in their environment. You will see why safety matters and how it is the key to assisting teens to let down their guard, relax their rigid defenses, and become willing to participate in activities with others. You will learn to read specific behaviors as expressions of unmet needs and unhealed trauma symptoms. You will get a basic understanding of the biology of the brain to understand how the brain plays a big part in why youth may have difficulty regulating their emotions. Most importantly, you will learn some practical tools to help teens transform their behavior by **creating safe environments, repairing ruptured relationships,** and helping them learn to **regulate their nervous systems**.

But before we explore these concepts, we must look at how adolescents view the world.

Teenagers generally think in an all-or-nothing way. Everything is black or white, good or bad, wonderful or awful. They love and hate you; you are their friend or enemy. Life is great; the world is terrible. This behavior is a natural part of this developmental stage, and understanding it may help you avoid personalizing it.

Teens who have experienced trauma from neglect or abuse may react to a variety of situations much more strongly than other adolescents. Much of their day is spent responding as if they are still under threat, and their behavior is primed for self-protection. They often remain hyperalert most of the day, ensuring nothing bad happens to them. It must be exhausting!

Teens with chronic trauma often feel a lack of control over their decisions because they were or still are thwarted or punished for them. As a result, they feel apathetic and often feel a lack of control over their lives.

This causes them to feel helpless and hopeless, anxious, or depressed. Teens who have experienced chronic trauma tend to isolate themselves from others because of deep feelings of shame, a lack of trust in others, and internal feelings of distress. It's difficult for these youth to form meaningful relationships with others because of a lack of trust and broken attachments by significant adults. They would rather be left alone. They can be highly defensive and resistant, especially with adults who, perhaps because of their own unhealed traumas, become reactive, making matters worse.

We can learn how to reach these teens by being a healing force in their lives. We can do this by learning to read reactive behavior as an expression of underlying distressing emotions, building trusting relationships and repairing them as needed, and setting up environments where teens feel safe and protected.

Teens who experience chronic trauma usually live in one of two chronic states, or cycle between them. The first state is **hyperarousal**, a feeling of overwhelm and even panic that interferes with their daily lives. The other condition is called **hypoarousal**, a reaction to trauma that results in feeling numb or "dead inside" and disconnected from the world. Understanding these conditions and other trauma reactions driven by internal distress can help us begin to read behavior as a signal for help and remove any preconceived labels or judgments. With this trauma-informed lens, we can understand that their behavior is a survival reaction and take steps to help teens feel safe and understood.

It's important to understand that after a trauma, the brain and body respond as if the danger is still there. The symptoms represent how teens have adapted to survive. They will become activated by unconscious triggers of the original trauma. The behavior is compensation for unresolved trauma and a defense against it. Symptoms of hyperarousal and hypoarousal are the most common symptoms of unhealed trauma.

Common Symptoms of Unhealed Trauma

Signs of chronic hyperarousal	Signs of chronic hypoarousal	Some other signs of unresolved trauma
• Restlessness • Jumpy, fidgety • Hyperactive • Always being on guard • Feeling unsafe • Difficulty relaxing • Impulsivity • Muscular tension (seen in their postures and gestures)	• Difficulty moving • Disconnected • Apathetic • Lethargic • Numb • Collapse/fainting • Slow or shallow breathing	• Denial (a defense used to deny a truth) • Dissociation (emotional detachment) • Avoidance (avoiding people, places or things) • Fight/flight response (body/mind preparation for escape or fight) • Shame • Intense mood swings

Take a few moments to review these symptoms and reflect on situations in which you may have encountered youth with these trauma reactions. Was it in a classroom, youth program, or other context?

It's important to understand that when an adolescent is exposed to danger at an early age, their brains change, and they are less likely to be able to manage their stressors than youth who did not have the early exposure. Their reactions are not just psychological; they are biological. The reaction is caused by a physical state, not a psychological response. You may find it helpful to understand that when individuals feel overwhelmed, parts of the brain shut down and other parts take over, making it impossible for them to self-regulate by thinking things through. It is a fascinating process that has been studied with the help of advances in science, such as functional magnetic resonance imaging (fMRIs). Let's learn about how the brain works, particularly when responding to overwhelming stress.

The Biology of the Brain

Those who research trauma are now recognizing that more than words are needed for healing. Many now believe that only through body-mind modalities, such as drama therapy and other creative arts approaches, can parts of the brain come into harmony.

To truly understand trauma responses, we need to understand the biology of the brain structure and how the brain responds to trauma. The brain has three layers: the cortex, the subcortical region, and the brain stem. Each is responsible for a different function.

The Cortex ("The Thinking Brain")

The cortex is the most sophisticated part of the brain and is responsible for higher mental functions. It can be considered the thinking brain and does not have much effect on our emotions or impulses. It is responsible for reasoning, problem-solving, verbal expression, and memories. This part of the brain can make decisions, process information, and explore possibilities.

The Limbic System ("The Emotional Brain" or "The Mammalian Brain")

The mammalian brain, or emotional brain, is responsible for feelings and memory but does not have words. It is responsible for nonverbal emotional experiences, feelings, and memories, including traumatic memories.

An important part of the limbic system is a small almond-shaped structure on either side of the head called **the amygdala,** detector of emotional memory. When a person is exposed to a threat, the amygdala activates, which generally triggers the "fight or flight" response. The amygdala is like a smoke detector, preparing us for danger.

The Brainstem ("The Reptilian Brain")

The reptilian brain governs our instincts, ensures our survival, and is the most primitive part of the brain. It controls our physiology and automatic responses such as heart rate and breathing. The reptilian brain has no language and stores emotional memories, including attachment experiences.[1]

Sometimes, one part of the brain takes over, pushing the other parts out of the way. For example, we may feel intense emotions that we just can't put words to. Or we can't control our impulses and actions, even when we want to. This is because our "thinking brain" is overridden by what is happening in our "emotional brain." The amygdala is the main controller of fear and anxiety. When it is activated, it shuts down the thinking brain so that we can react instinctively to danger, which can be a good thing, and sometimes even lifesaving. But sometimes it is a false alarm.

Teens who have experienced developmental trauma may have an overactive amygdala. They can be triggered by a sound, a word, a person, or something else that taps into a traumatic memory or feeling. They go into an automatic trauma response, such as fight or flight. This response may seem extreme or aggressive and can translate into what some adults call "acting-out behavior."

A triggered response can be instinctive and become highly aggressive or even violent. In these moments, the thinking brain shuts off and is unavailable. It is not until an individual calms down that the thinking brain comes back online. It is difficult to talk a person down during this time. Asking them to stop and breathe is the main thing that can help. Conversely, there are times when teens, or anyone else, can think logically but cannot feel it. This time, the thinking brain overrides the emotional brain, pushing away upsetting feelings. The goal is to coordinate the parts of the brain so that neither the feeling brain nor the thinking brain takes over to the exclusion of the other.

A safe environment is essential to teens who have experienced trauma. If they inaccurately perceive their current environment as dangerous, based on past unsafe experiences (their nervous system is routinely on high alert), they can go into a reactive trauma response. This is why it is essential for teachers and others working with youth to create safe physical and emotional spaces.

Neuroception: The Safe-Environment Scanning System

When treating trauma, nothing is more important than safety. Individuals naturally respond to what feels safe and unsafe in their environment. They do so in an automatic, unconscious process called neuroception, a term coined by Dr. Stephen Porges. Individuals who have experienced trauma develop **faulty neuroception,** an inability to perceive the environment or the people in it as safe and trustworthy.

Porges explains that the brain does not differentiate between real or imagined danger. When someone has experienced early trauma, they are likely to miscalculate the environmental risk factor. They may feel unsafe, anxious, and frightened even in safe, peaceful environments. As a result of faulty neuroception, the nervous system kicks into high gear, placing an individual on high alert, ready to defend. In this heightened state, the individual is easily triggered. This can explain the reactivity in some of our youth. They are reacting to what they feel is unsafe.

When teaching a class or leading an activity, you may have experienced a student becoming easily triggered for what seemed like no apparent reason; perhaps it was a look or a sound that caused them to react and lash out. Something caused them to feel unsafe. The look may have reminded them of an unsafe person in their lives, or they may have had an old body memory while doing the activity. Vulnerable youth will view anything or anyone that triggers the emergence of unsafe feelings as the enemy and will react as a survival mechanism to protect themselves. They are on high alert, and they are ready to defend.

A vulnerable or dysregulated nervous system caused by trauma makes it difficult for a teen to return to a calmer state. Unless the issue is addressed by an understanding adult or peer who can help calm them down so they feel protected, teens can spiral out of control, unaware of what they are experiencing. In many cases, their behavior is an involuntary response to what they believe is a threat. Once triggered, they may become reactive, leading to extreme reactions, engaging in conflicts, and even resorting to violence.

Those of us who work with youth who have experienced trauma can greatly benefit from preparing for the effects of neuroception. We can create safe, contained classroom environments and other supportive peer programs. In Chapter 7, I discuss how the ENACT Method implements a "creative container," developed to provide a safe space where creativity is encouraged.

Based on Porges' theory of neuroception, we can understand what happens when a dysregulated youth returns to a more balanced state when they feel safe and calm. I can recall a student I'll call Roger. After being triggered by something said by a peer, Roger was yelling and threatening the other student in the hallway. In the following class period, I saw Roger smiling and laughing with his peers in an ENACT workshop. At first glance, when I observed him participating in the workshop, I wasn't even sure it was Roger, the threatening, dysregulated student I had seen less than an hour earlier. The emotionally protective environment set up by the ENACT instructors allowed him to relax his defenses so he could return to being himself.

The following two concepts, HALT and the Window of Tolerance, are not necessarily symptoms of developmental trauma. But they are useful concepts to know because they can explain what may have contributed to Roger's triggering. They can also be applied universally.

HALT and the Window of Tolerance

HALT is an acronym for Hunger, Anger, Loneliness, and Tiredness.[2] When teens experience any one of these conditions, they are more likely to struggle with their physical and emotional health, leading them to become more easily triggered.

For example, if someone is hungry, their blood sugar can get low, and they can become irritable. *Hunger* can create mood swings. Impulse control is affected. If someone is *angry,* they can experience negative emotions affecting their perceptions and decision-making skills. *Loneliness* can lead to isolation, causing more loneliness, which can lead to depression and ultimately generate poor decisions and reactive behavior. If they are *tired* because they stayed up all night and did not get a good night's sleep, their emotions will be affected. The next day, they may be more likely to engage in negative thinking and engage in conflicts with others. And, of course, if more than one condition occurs, the problems increase.

The Window of Tolerance is a concept that explains why a person may become quickly and easily frustrated. It describes the range of arousal levels at which a person can handle stress. Dr. Daniel Siegel, a clinical professor of psychiatry, explains in his book *Mindsight* that our windows of tolerance determine how comfortable we feel with specific memories, issues, emotions, and physical sensations. He explains, "Within our window of tolerance, we remain receptive; outside of it, we become reactive."[3] When the window is wide, it helps us handle stress. When it is narrow, our tolerance level is small and can lead to negative feelings and choices.

This concept does not apply just to youth, of course. We, too, have our windows of tolerance, and we can observe them in other adults as well. For those of us who work in schools, hospitals, community centers, etc., it is hard to ignore the staff's frustration level and reactive behavior when dealing with dysregulated teens. This level of frustration can be due to their narrowing window of tolerance, when they often don't have the time to recalibrate. This window can become more and more narrow until sometimes it is completely shut.

After sessions with students, some of my ENACT staff complained about the lack of patience they saw from the teachers in their classrooms. But my teaching artists were visitors for only a limited time, brief enough for them to stay within their window of tolerance. Exhausted teachers must endure stress all day, with little downtime and likely too many responsibilities. Teachers' levels of stress and frustration can run high, and without self-care can unintentionally lead to their own reactive behavior. They often don't have the bandwidth they need to manage their anxiety triggered by reactive youth, let alone manage the stress of others.

We can learn to read our internal signals and try to learn how and when to self-regulate so our window widens. In those moments when frustration is building, it is helpful to realize we are reaching our peak of tolerance and to find a way to give ourselves space to regulate, even for a few moments. For those living or working with youth, understanding their window of tolerance and your own can help you know how to relate best to them—including stepping back when necessary.

To summarize, symptoms of trauma stay with an individual long after the actual traumatic event occurs. Body memories can trigger feelings of fear, and external factors, like sounds or unexpected movements, can cause someone with trauma to leap into survival mode, compelled to defend themselves. These are reactive symptoms of someone trying to survive even though a real threat is not currently present.

The next chapter will outline what happens to teens in the aftermath of trauma and offer suggestions on how to help them heal.

Below is the rest of the case history of Michelle, the sarcastic and cautious teen, that was introduced at the start of this chapter.

———————

My teaching partner, Jason, explained to the class that we were there to teach them some acting skills and that we would demonstrate a few techniques to see if they were interested. "We're the bad kids, right?" said the girl named "I don't know," repeating a question I heard often when meeting a new group of teens. "That's why we were picked, right?"

No wonder she didn't trust me, I thought. The girl assumed I had arrived expecting them to play the part of "bad kids acting out," and she did not miss her cue. "I don't know" was the line of the natural performer. I explained that we were asked to be there to work with them because some kids had trouble managing their behavior. I told her I had found that kids with "behavior problems" are the best actors and actresses and that I wasn't kidding.

"I want to try to develop that acting talent," I said, "but we all have a choice to be here." I encouraged the girls to try out the drama group that I was proposing and see if each of them was honestly interested in being a part of it.

Nine of the 12 students chose to participate with the group for the next two weeks; the others preferred to sit in the back with the teacher. Later in the week, after observing the activities and their peers enjoying themselves, the others joined in, although some were reluctant. Aware of their resistance, we needed to help them build a sense of trust with us and each other. We all created and signed a contract of agreement that spelled out guidelines for support and encouragement. The group chose the consequences (which were never punitive) if the contract were to be broken. This usually involved stepping out of the group activity until they felt they could support each other.

Unison theater games would be an engaging start to the group process, with just enough challenge to avoid them feeling infantilized; that would be a deal breaker. As trust was developed, my partner and I moved on to a deeper phase. I wanted to help them reflect on their defensive behavior and discover what they were protecting.

Standing in a circle, I introduced an attitude game. I told them that this exercise would be easy for them because they were good actors. "On the count of three, I said, put on the biggest, coolest attitude pose you can. Show the expression on your face and your body. One, two, three! Strike a pose!" The students embodied their attitude poses and then wore their defensive facial masks. "Now exaggerate your poses," I said. I heard laughter as the students embellished their poses. Some had clenched fists; others had their hands up with their palms facing out as if saying, "Stay away from me," a pose I was quite familiar with. I had seen others touching their waists, leaning broadly into one hip. "Freeze," I directed them to look at the other adolescents around the room. They giggled as they observed each other's poses. "Unfreeze," I said, asking them what their body felt like in this pose. Were their muscles tight? Did they feel rigid or frozen? I could see them contemplating.

I went around the circle and tapped some of them on the shoulder, asking them to tell me what their attitude was. "How do you feel?" I asked the first student. "Angry," she said, snarling at me. I walked over to another student and tapped her on the shoulder. "What are you thinking?" "I wish I didn't have to be in school today. I hate it here." Finally, I walked over to the "I don't know" girl and asked, "Is there something you want to say? "Yes," she replied. "Please leave me alone! Everyone is always on my case, and I'm sick of it. I want to be left alone!" "Got it," I replied and moved on. We directed the students to take a deep breath and relax their faces, hands, chest, and stomach muscles. They were invited to tune in to their bodies after that. "Relaxed," a student said, and several nodded in agreement. I eyed the "I don't know" girl. She was nodding her head in agreement.

These adolescents transformed from looking hardened, cold, and unapproachable to being open and available. As they looked around the room at each other's faces, they acknowledged the change they felt. One student explained how connected she felt to the others in the group. Once back in their seats, the "I don't know" girl raised her hand. "My real name is Michelle," she declared. "Nice to meet you, Michelle," I said and smiled. It was as if we both quietly understood something had changed.

We talked about various attitudes, poses, and roles they said they observed in school and in their community. They reflected on their own. I explained to them how they could put on attitudes anytime and remove them when they wanted to. "You own the pose. The pose doesn't own you," I explained.

"Which pose was easier?" I asked. "The attitude pose or the relaxed one?"

"The attitude pose," Michelle responded. Most agreed.

"Really? Why is that?"

"We are not used to being relaxed; it makes us nervous. It makes us feel scared," another adolescent added. This hit me with a sad clarity. It was a reminder that individuals who experienced trauma feel they always need to stay on guard for potential danger. It's difficult for them to relax. For these youth, attitudes were their form of protection.

As the exercise was concluding, a student raised their hand and said, "I liked it because I could connect better to the others in the circle." This confirmed to me that being part of a supportive group gives youth the safety they need to drop their guard, at least temporarily. These adolescents were more comfortable maintaining their defenses than releasing them. They held onto them for dear life, and it kept them stuck in a role. Their pose was their body armor. Their badge of honor was their attitude, protecting them from feeling vulnerable. It would take time for them to discover new tools to replace the defenses, but eventually they learned to find their voice and connect to their authenticity.

Case History Notes

- At times, teens do not trust adults. This is understandable in youth who have been lied to, harmed, betrayed, or abandoned by adults. Even when teens are not coming from dire circumstances, adolescence is often a time when they question adult authority.
- Teens develop "attitudes" as a coping mechanism to protect their vulnerable parts.

The goal is to establish trust with teens who are highly resistant.

Techniques I use include:

- Developing mutual respect by agreeing on reciprocal boundaries.
- Finding something to agree upon.
- Finding something that you can authentically praise.
- Attuning with youth by validating their opinions and feelings.

In the final phase of the attitude exercise, I asked the teens to relax their faces, arms, and chests. They were learning to let go of their rigid postures and to explore a grounded, centered place. We all breathed together. When I asked them to reflect on their feelings, one student said, "I feel connected to myself and everyone in the group."

Notes

1 Fisher, *The Living Legacy of Trauma Flip Chart*.
2 This acronym comes from Alcoholics Anonymous.
3 Siegel, *Mindsight*, 137.

Chapter 3

The Aftermath of Developmental Trauma

The story begins when a high school principal tells us about Wendy, a lovely, shy young person who has been a victim of severe bullying since she was a child. Wendy was in the ENACT Dropout Prevention Program, designed for students at risk of dropping out of school because they missed over 50 days in a year. Her class was selected to participate in this program for a full year as part of a citywide initiative to significantly increase attendance.

ENACT would work with the students to create a public performance for those who missed no more than three sessions each semester. The audience would include friends, family, teachers, and other supportive staff. Students would work with ENACT actors daily on the issues that prevented them from coming to school. The show's theme was based on issues they wanted to tackle, such as violence, peer pressure, and cyberbullying, which were often suggested. Each class voted on the theme.

On the first day I arrived, Wendy sat quietly at her desk and way back into the corner of the room. Until then, Wendy had not participated in any group theater games or role-play activities. But when ideas for a theme were thrown around, and cyberbullying was an option, Wendy's hand flew up. She joined the voting process, and cyberbullying was the winning theme.

At the beginning of the second week, I approached Wendy, asking her why she sat alone and never participated with the other students. She looked at me as if she were trying to figure me out, and said, "I was bullied so much growing up that now I just keep to myself. I feel safer that way. I was teased for years for being fat,

DOI: 10.4324/9781003415022-5

and I'm still overweight, so I sit by myself, and this way, no one bothers me."

I asked her to tell me more. She would tell me a story that would break my heart.

Developmental trauma, also known as chronic trauma, has a significant impact on the lives of adolescents, with effects that can be long-lasting. Wendy, who was stuck in a role I call The Victim, suffered from chronic trauma. You can read the rest of her case history at the end of this chapter.

Most teens who grow up with early trauma learn to adapt to their environment, but at a cost. They may live in a state of chronic hyperarousal, always on the lookout for danger. Their behavior becomes a defense against internal and external stress and danger. These teens are hungry for acceptance and love from their caregivers, but if their needs are unmet, they often grow to believe they are unworthy of love. They live with a deep hole that can't be filled. They may develop negative self-concepts and experience self-blame and guilt. They often feel powerless and hopeless and believe others are not to be trusted. Teens who grow up in environments with emotional or physical danger often have generalized perceptions of the world that are not true in their present environment. These perceptions may lead them to believe that people want to hurt them and that they are not safe.

Triggers

Growing up in environments where there was verbal abuse or neglect, teens become highly sensitive to other people and their behaviors. Perceived threats can cause them to react with immediate and extreme behaviors. A situation or event can activate their suppressed feelings, and the emergence of these feelings is scary and difficult for them to manage. This activation is a cue for danger, called a **trigger.** Triggers cause the emergence of suppressed emotions.

Among teens who have experienced developmental trauma, certain actions, looks, or behaviors can trigger feelings including, but not limited to, the following:

- Feeling disrespected.
- Feeling ignored.

- Feeling shamed.
- Feeling threatened.
- Feeling powerless.
- Feeling afraid.
- Feeling unseen.
- Feeling needs were not met.
- Feeling targeted.

Triggers can evoke a body memory or tap unwanted feelings. Let's say that a student named John blew off his homework. When a teacher tells John to stay after class to finish his assignments, he feels attacked, and anger swells up. He is sure the teacher is shaming him in front of the class. John is triggered.

John's assumptions were based on his history of growing up in a home where he was neglected and shamed in front of his family. To John, adults are untrustworthy and can hurt him.

If you are a teacher or a youth worker, I am sure you have seen youth become triggered. Can you recall instances when your students became triggered?

Behavioral Responses

Behavioral responses are reactions to triggers. When John, from the example above, is triggered, he is likely to have a strong behavioral response—such as fight or flight—and might slam down his books and run out of the room.

Youth who have experienced developmental trauma are always looking for safety. They develop behaviors as survival mechanisms and create defenses as adaptations to their home environment. If they grew up with chronic neglect or abuse, if they experience or witness extreme violence, these youth need to find ways to survive. To keep themselves out of danger, they often remain in a state of hypervigilance.

But what if real danger is not present in their current environments, such as school classrooms or auditoriums? Unfortunately, a part of their brain may not recognize the difference between real and perceived danger and activates the body to respond any time the perceived danger is present. Adults such as teachers and youth workers need to understand where the behavior comes from to help the student rather than reprimand or punish them.

Common Trigger Responses

These include three common categories of trauma responses—fight, flight, and freeze.[1]

Fight: Physiological arousal

- Aggression.
- Irritability/anger.
- Trouble concentrating.
- Hyperactivity or "silliness".

Flight: Withdrawal and escape

- Social isolation.
- Avoidance of others.
- Sitting alone in class or at recess.
- Running away.

Freeze: Stilling and constriction

- Constricted emotional expression.
- Stilling of behavior.
- Over-compliance and denial of needs.

Have you observed the above behavioral responses in the teens you know? Is it a habitual behavior, or does it happen under certain circumstances? How have you handled it in the past? Would this new information change your perception about youths' behavior?

In Chapter 1, we discussed that if caregivers have not met children's emotional and physical needs during a critical time in early development, those children will be significantly affected. These caregivers are not "bad people"; they may have failed to attend to their child's needs for deep-seated reasons, including substance abuse or mental illness. In cases like these, children may feel alone when navigating their emotions. They lack important tools. Without an adult to help them manage their feelings, they often cannot self-regulate and may develop a negative self-concept. These youth may go to great lengths to seek attention and love from others because, in a sense, they feel parentless. They may act very needy and seek attention constantly.

Everyday Emotional Needs[2]

Underlying needs

- Emotionally demanding behavior (whiny, interrupting, dramatic).
- Seeking negative attention (acting out).
- Poor interpersonal boundaries (e.g., too much sharing).
- Attempts to control the environment may be described as "lying" or manipulative.

Physical needs

- Physical nurturance-seeking behavior (e.g., too much physical contact, poor physical boundaries, sexual behaviors).
- Hoarding or stealing food, clothing, and objects.

When have you seen any of these behaviors in the teens you work with?

The Body's Response to Trauma

Trauma expert Dr. Peter Levine explains that trauma is stored in the body and that "the 'triggering' event itself does not cause trauma symptoms. They stem from the frozen residue of energy that has not been resolved and discharged. This residue remains trapped in the nervous system where it can wreak havoc on our bodies and spirits."[3]

In other words, the initial trauma lasts way beyond the traumatic event itself and can live in our bodies for years unless it is addressed. For youth and others, the effects of trauma keep them in a state of hypervigilance (always on the lookout for danger) and is a **defensive reaction** that can be misunderstood as hyperactivity.

Pat Ogden, PhD, a leader in somatic (body-centered) approaches to psychotherapy, explains that certain behaviors are what she calls "body responses." In her book *Trauma and the Body*, she says, "impulses for fight behavior are often experienced somatically by clients as tension in the hands, arms, shoulders; hands beginning to tighten or curl into a fist; lifting of the hand or arms; narrowing of the eyes; clenching of the jaw; impulses to kick or struggle."[4] This describes the aggressive, "acting-out students" my team and I encountered in the schools where we were invited to work. In Chapter 8, you will read about how ENACT actors take on these behaviors in their role portrayal and mirror them back to the students so they can gain perspective.

Ogden lists certain compliant, submissive behaviors as trauma reactions as well. These include "crouching, ducking the head, avoiding eye contact, bowing the back before the perpetrator and generally appearing physically smaller and consequently less noticeable and threatening."[5] This clearly describes the students we encountered who were labeled as "withdrawn." These postures, gestures, and facial expressions were indications of trauma!

To summarize, when the mind cannot process trauma, it is stored in the body, where it becomes stuck in armored defenses, appearing in posture, attitude, and facial expression. The body becomes a storehouse for unwanted thoughts and feelings in an attempt to push away emotional pain. The emotions may be suppressed but have not disappeared; they concretize in the body.

Adaptations

Teens with developmental trauma, especially those who have adverse or broken attachments with caregivers, rely on their behaviors to protect them from harm and from feeling distressing emotions. Unfortunately, many of these behaviors cause them to split off from their feelings, separating them from a full connection with themselves and from forming healthy relationships with others. Some of these behaviors are self-destructive, which causes additional challenges for them.

Common Behavioral Adaptations
Including taking on and getting stuck in a role[6]:

- Emotional numbing.
- Withdrawal/avoidance.
- Indiscriminate attachments.
- Hyper-control of environment/rigidity.
- Substance abuse.
- Alterations in eating patterns.
- Constricted or excessive sexual behaviors.
- Aggressive or other externalizing behaviors.

There are myriad other symptoms that may occur in the aftermath of trauma. Some are somatic (physical symptoms resulting from emotional distress), and others result in negative self-concept, developing false selves, and self-destructive behaviors.

Physical Complaints

"I don't feel well! Can I go to the nurse's office?"

This is a request teachers hear daily. Those of you who work in schools have often seen children in classrooms get sent to the nurse's office only to be returned to class, told there is nothing wrong with them. But something is wrong; they may have somaticized their unmanageable feelings because they do not have the resources to manage them.

I remember entering a classroom where students had just experienced a horrific event, a stabbing outside their school. When I came to work with them the next day, almost all of them complained of having headaches, nausea, and dizziness, which were clear signs of trauma. When they could finally voice their feelings about the trauma, they stopped having the symptoms. Youth need opportunities to externalize their emotions instead of suppressing them. (You can read more about this and other case histories about collective trauma in Appendices.)

Common Emotional Effects of Trauma

Shame

Perhaps the most common response to trauma is shame. Students have told me that being shamed, especially by an adult, feels like "someone punched you in the gut." It can lead to feelings of fear, anger, rage, and negative self-worth. Just as peers can provide lifelines of support to each other, they can also trigger devastating feelings of shame if an adolescent is embarrassed, cast out of the group or bullied. For some youth, shame is triggered by perceived criticism; for example, if they are called out for a mistake they made in the classroom. This is especially true if they grew up in households where they were belittled or neglected. For youth who grew up feeling unheard, humiliated, and belittled by caregivers, being shamed feels like that original trauma is happening all over again.

Children depend on their caregivers for needs, both basic and intangible, and are afraid of blaming them, making their already shaky lives feel even more out of control. Instead, they often blame themselves. Chronic shame prevents youth from forming and sustaining relationships with their peers in schools and other social settings. Shame often results in isolation, which is bad enough. But when coupled with other symptoms, it can feel so overwhelming that it creates additional symptoms of trauma.

Dissociation

When feelings or memories become too overwhelming to endure, adolescents can sometimes cut themselves off from their emotions, resulting in the perception of being "unreal" or numb. A young client of mine describes the experience as being in "nowhere land, where your feet are not on the ground, and you are somewhere out there, unable to find the boundaries around you." Others have described this state as spaciness, blankness, disconnection, or being split off from themselves and others. The term for this is **dissociation**, which Bessel van der Kolk calls "the essence of trauma."[7]

If you work with teens who have experienced trauma, you probably encounter forms of dissociation. Have you ever asked an adolescent what was bothering them, and their response was, "I don't know?" The more you push, the more they repeat the same answer and become increasingly resistant. I learned this the hard way with my client, Jenna.

An Example of Dissociation

Early in my private practice, I worked with a 16-year-old adolescent who was reportedly "oppositional" and labeled "unreachable." My first thought was, what was she protecting? Jenna, as I will call her, had a history of early attachment trauma, with a depressed mom and an absent dad. In her teens, she had been assaulted and raped more than once. She had turned to drinking and drugs and ended up cycling through several residential programs.

When Jenna arrived for our first session in mid-winter, she took off her coat, revealing only a black bra and a tight skirt underneath. Her eyes were painted with strong black Egyptian-looking liner, and her lips were colored bright pink. Each week she arrived in another creative and revealing outfit. Each week I pointed out how artistic she was. After the first few sessions, she brought in her portfolio. She loved to draw and take photographs, and she was quite talented. From then on, we started her session each week with her showing me something from her sketchbook.

Our relationship was developing, but whenever I asked her about her family, she made it clear to me right away that that topic was off limits. One day, I pushed too far and asked her about her relationship with her parents, and within seconds I watched her disappear. She continued to talk, but it was as if she was disconnected from her body. She went into a coma-like state for a few minutes, stared at her hands, and looked as though she were frozen. "Jenna, Jenna," I said. "Where are you?" After a few moments, she seemed to return to her body. "Where were you?" I asked. "I don't know. I forgot," she replied.

From that day on, I gained a new respect for the phenomenon of dissociation. I had seen such symptoms before, but not to this extreme. I came to believe that the more extreme the dissociation, the more extreme the trauma.

I would not ask Jenna about her family again for a long time, until we had worked on her symptoms. I knew it would take a long time to help Jenna connect with her emotions without her splitting off. There was no doubt we needed to work indirectly. Words were not enough. We would find other ways for her to express herself. We did guided meditations and breathing exercises, but I always put her in the driver's seat.

Jenna taught me how to draw. One day, Jenna began to sketch figures. They appeared to be variations of herself. She drew pictures of herself in different costumes and we discussed what it might feel like to wear those outfits, take them off, and try another.

Jenna surprised me when she arrived the next week. She wore plain blue jeans and a t-shirt, wearing little makeup. She seemed more relaxed and more at ease in her body. We talked about what it felt like to wear no makeup versus wearing a lot of it. The next week she brought her makeup in, and we both experimented with it.

Something was beginning to shift in Jenna. Her face was softer, her body seemed less armored, and she appeared comfortable with herself. I asked her if we could make the figures she drew "come to life" by creating statues of them with our bodies. She pointed to the figure she wanted to embody and told me which one I should take on. One day, she embodied the role of a figure with a lot of makeup and a sparse outfit. "Freeze," I said.

After I had her shake off the exercise, I asked her what it felt like to be stuck in only one role. "Not good," she answered. "It's more fun to play them all." Jenna learned she could be more than the limited role she placed on herself.

Secrets and Lies: Holding on to Control

The need for privacy and secret-keeping is not unusual for adolescents; it is part of the developmental period when they discover and define their boundaries. However, adolescents with chronic trauma have an additional reason for keeping their cards close to their chests. If they feel that there is no hope in life and nothing will change, they keep secrets, afraid others will find out. Children and teens who experience neglect or abuse in their homes are often afraid to talk about themselves to people outside of their homes because they believe it could lead to their caregivers getting into trouble, or they fear they could be removed from their homes and placed in foster care. These young people suffer terrible inner turmoil. Instead of telling others about their situations and seeking help, they hide it. They isolate, deny their feelings, and are highly resistant to being exposed. Others will lie about their home situations because they are terrified their secret may be revealed.

Youth behavior is an expression of their internal lives. When teens hide their feelings, keeping them secret tells us something is wrong. Understanding youth behavior as a language of its own is a worthy act. You will gain valuable insight so you can respond compassionately while seeking ways to help them. This is what leads to genuine connection and healing. This is the first step in letting them know you care and that they are not alone. And of course, if you suspect abuse, find out who you can report to who is trained and qualified in this area.

Loss of Dignity

In my work in New York City's schools, I observed how hurtful it is to teens when they feel disrespected or insulted by their peers or teachers. They feel their dignity is undermined, and this, to them, is a significant offense, especially true for those who grew up with a history of neglect and abuse. If adolescents are devalued by their caregivers, being shamed, ignored, or worse, their already shaky self-concept is damaged again. A feeling of a loss of dignity caused by someone else can trigger them to have the same painful feelings all over again. If they were too afraid or unable to speak up, their bottled-up feelings could emerge through their behavior, sometimes with a vengeance.

The media often covers stories about the fallout of rageful youth retaliation. If teens grow up witnessing fighting and violence, whether it is among their peers, by family members, or by police, this is behavior they may end up imitating. They likely will seek retaliation in defense of their self-worth, and their anger can escalate to rage. It can be shocking how some youth will stand up for their dignity, but once rage is let loose, it can be impossible to contain. This is why it is critical to help youth see their self-worth and manage their emotions before a situation gets out of control.

Learning and Behavioral Challenges

When trauma reactions interfere with or distract students from learning, they can often be mistaken for learning disabilities.[8] A youth's lack of ability to concentrate or their tendency to become easily distracted can lead them to be misunderstood and pinned with a learning or behavioral label, which, unfortunately, they are likely to internalize.

For example, "Jose" may look out the window during class, appear uninterested in his work, and act "spacy." Further investigation reveals that despite repeated requests from the teacher to stay focused, Jose is **dissociating** (being detached from himself and those around him) and is looking out the window to avoid thinking about his complicated feelings.

"Michael" constantly glances around the room and frequently gets up from his desk. His teacher tells him to sit down, but he is up again in moments, scanning the room. After several attempts to keep Michael in his seat, the teacher reports that he is "hyperactive." Further investigation reveals that Michael is hypervigilant (on guard for danger) because of his developmental trauma growing up in an unsafe home. Michael learned to stay on guard from an early age to protect himself from harm.

Trauma symptoms can mimic symptoms of hyperactivity or attention-deficit/hyperactivity disorder (ADHD). While a teen with trauma may be diagnosed with ADHD, this diagnosis has limited use without identifying the cause.[9] It is unfortunate how often teachers and other well-meaning adults who work with children look for an immediate solution for a student's learning difficulty and overlook the possibility that they may be suffering from trauma.

Substance Abuse

Many teens experiment with alcohol and drugs. This can be a way for them to fit in with peers or to manage their emotions. However, experimentation can become a problem if a teen has a genetic disposition to substance abuse, or if drinking or using another substance leads to risky behavior or becomes a habit.

Teens may use substances as a way to soothe anxiety or as a way of emotional numbing. But on a deeper level, substance abuse can fill an emotional void for teens with negative attachment histories. As Gabor Mate explains, "Addiction is a complex psychological, emotional, physiological, neurobiological, social and spiritual process. It manifests through any behavior in which a person finds temporary relief or pleasure."[10]

How can we help teens fill that void in more positive ways? It is possible if a caring adult, such as a teacher, a coach, or a neighbor, can build meaningful relationships with them, and whenever possible, aim to heal broken attachments. Caring adults who form and maintain meaningful attachments with teens can help them avoid self-soothing addictions.

Bullying

In 2012, the World Health Organization reported that one-third of children worldwide have been bullied by their peers. Chronic bullying is characterized by threatening behavior that can include name-calling, teasing, making faces, or hitting. The Youth Bullying Prevention Act, passed in 2012, required schools to implement comprehensive anti-bullying policies. And yet, in 2019, about 22 percent of students ages 12–18 still reported being bullied at school.[11]

Clinical psychologist Gorden Neufeld, PhD, says bullying entails "a significant loss of feeling as the young brain's defensive apparatus becomes stuck to defend...against a sense of vulnerability that is too overwhelming."[12]

Put more simply, bullies are often trying to avoid feelings of vulnerability. Bullies need to be in control because they so often feel out of control. They are easily triggered. Seeing others as vulnerable enrages them because it reminds them of their own feelings of vulnerability, which they have worked so hard to defend. They may bully to address or eliminate the threat, enhancing their sense of being in control, however misguided.

But bullying doesn't bring these teens what they truly crave: a sense of attachment. We discussed earlier that youth without the experience of proper attachment with a caregiver are at a terrible disadvantage because they must learn to manage emotions on their own, without guidance. And they generally have trouble doing so because they were never taught the appropriate tools for self-regulation. The tools they use—vicious attacks—are dangerous to others and themselves. With their protruding jaws and armored postures, bullies are prime examples of youth who are stuck in a role. They show us their tough façades of hardened emotions that tell us, if we know how to read them, how vulnerable they truly are.

Self-Injury

Mary Pipher, the author of the beautiful book *Reviving Ophelia*, says that self-injury is like "psychic pain turned inward in the most physical way."[13] Self-harm, such as cutting or burning, is an unhealthy coping strategy some youth use to relieve their emotional pain or to help them self-regulate. Sometimes, they use it to manage big feelings like anger that have turned inward. Adults need to understand that inflicting self-harm does not necessarily mean that a teen is suicidal. Self-harm is nearly always a temporary relief of unbearable feelings. Of course, evidence of self-harm is frightening for adults when they discover it. This habitual behavior needs to be addressed as soon as possible, but we may not be able to help them immediately and we need to have patience as we teach them more positive coping skills to manage painful emotions. Again, forming meaningful attachments with teens is an important element for their healing.

Sarah: Overcoming Self-Injury

I worked with 16-year-old Sarah in my private practice. When she first arrived at my office, she wore an oversized sweatshirt with long sleeves covering her arms. Her social worker had told me that she had been cutting herself for close to a year and was unwilling to talk to her about her feelings. Sarah had been sent to me because she loved acting, and her social worker hoped we could address her issues through role-play. We played theater games for the first few sessions as I built a relationship with her.

During the games, Sarah kept criticizing herself, saying things like, "I'm stupid," "I can't do this," and "I hate myself." One day, I asked her when she started saying hurtful things about herself. She told me that she had been blaming herself ever since her mom left her when she was six. "Do you think it is your fault that she left?"

"Yes," she said, "I was too much for her."

"All kids are too much," I said, and we laughed together. "I would guess your mom had other problems, too, right?"

I knew her mom had substance abuse problems, and that was why Sarah was taken out of the house and placed into foster care. We had a lot of work to do. I understood it would be a long process because Sarah had lost her early attachment to her mom, which I am sure started long before she was taken out of the house.

"I know you like acting," I said. "Are there any TV shows or movies you like?"

Sarah immediately talked about a television show she was watching that revolved around a group of high school students and their trials and tribulations. "Let's look for some monologues from that show." She was excited.

"You know, actors need to learn to deal with all kinds of feelings to perform them on television and the stage. How do you know when people are dealing with challenging feelings?" I asked.

Sarah suddenly pulled up her sleeves and showed me her cuts. "This is how I deal with mine," she said. "It makes me feel better. It helps me calm down when I'm upset."

I thanked her for being so honest. I understood that Sarah had a lot of emotional pain and that cutting was her only way of dealing with it. She did not have other skills to cope with her emotions. She likely never learned to self-regulate and self-soothe at an early age because she didn't have a caregiver to soothe her.

Over the next few months, we worked on monologues to help Sarah express herself and practiced coping skills like self-talk, breathing, and tapping to help her self-soothe. She was developing acting skills and self-regulation skills at the same time. She opened up about her feelings as her cutting lessened each week. She pulled up her sleeve one week and said, "Look, I didn't cut this week."

To summarize, youth who cut and self-mutilate are not trying to commit suicide. They are using cutting as a coping tool to manage their difficult emotions because they do not have more positive coping skills. We can help these youth learn the tools to deal with their feelings.

Suicide Attempts: Attacks on the Self

Distinct from teens who inflict self-harm, some teens do attempt to kill themselves. Suicide threats should never be dismissed as attention-seeking or dramatic. As of this writing, suicide is the second leading cause of death for children, adolescents, and young adults aged 15–24.[14]

There are many reasons why a teen may feel suicidal. Pressures at school, societal strains, depression, anxiety, unhealed substance abuse, and bullying, both in person and via social media, have led children to take their own lives. And it is not just those who are bullied who are drawn to suicide but also the bullies themselves.

Peer pressure, too, can be a major strain on young lives. The isolation can be devastating when youth fail to fit in and are rejected by their peers. We have discussed how essential peer groups are to teens, especially to those who suffer from neglect or abuse. Sometimes, peer groups are a teen's only source of support. Losing that support can be unbearable, and it is extreme enough for them to feel they can't go on.

A lack of support can be especially crushing for gay, lesbian, and trans youth, who may also feel devalued by family members or society at large. The Trevor Project 2023 U.S. National Survey on Mental Health of LGBTQ youth found that 41% of young people seriously considered attempting suicide in the past year, including roughly half of the transgender and nonbinary youth who responded. These teens often feel isolated and struggle alone. Some cover up how they feel. They create roles out of fear of being exposed. They may internalize the feelings of hatred and turn it in on themselves.

What if a teen is having thoughts of suicide and there is no one to talk to? What if they do not feel someone on their side is rooting for them? What if they feel there is no way out? It is critical for caring adults to be there for struggling youth, and if there is concern about suicide, to get them the professional help they need as soon as possible.

Below you'll find the rest of the story that began at the start of this chapter. It shows a young teen's brave struggle with thoughts of suicide and describes her transformation.

———————

"When I was little," Wendy said in a quiet voice, "kids at school would gang up on me and push me into a corner, and I couldn't get out. 'You are fat, you are fat,' they would yell. They would laugh at me, tease me, and pull my hair. Then, when I was in third grade, I started being badly bullied at school because I was fat, and it never stopped. I was bullied so much that I began to hate myself."

Wendy explained that despite being kind and supportive, her mother could not stop the bullying. She was a busy single working mom. Wendy didn't want to upset her mom by telling her details about her torment, so she tried to hide her feelings. She would sit in her room and write poems. When she finally confided in her mom, her mom was again supportive; she responded with advice and went to the school several times to complain.

But nothing changed. Wendy continued to be bullied every day. She began to come late to school or not show up at all. This accounted for her poor attendance record. Her mother's love was just not enough to spare her from her devastating emotional pain.

Wendy looked down at the floor and described what happened next. Unable to deal with the pain, she attempted to end her life. Just in time, her mom found her with a knife in her hand and stopped her. She called an ambulance, and Wendy was immediately hospitalized and sent home a few days later with medicine.

But medicine can't stop bullying. When Wendy returned to school, she was bullied again. "Ever since then," she said, "I stay to myself, so no one bothers me." We sat in silence together, and then I had an idea: Her story might help others.

We talked about how her bullying experience might be incorporated into the upcoming yearly ENACT theater performance that her class was developing and would offer a valuable message. She did not need to share her personal story; I thought it safer if someone else could act as her voice. Wendy agreed without hesitation.

Wendy began participating in the group, and her peers immediately accepted her. She played theater games and participated in role-plays that addressed bullying. "I write rhythms and poetry," she told us one day. To my surprise, she shared her excitement about creating a rap about bullying, an "anti-bully rap theme song." When I returned to the class the next week, I saw Wendy teaching the song to two of her classmates, her backup singers. Her confidence was growing by leaps and bounds.

As we approached the performance date, each participant was asked if they had a message they wanted to share with the audience that might help them understand the growing cyberbullying problem.

Wendy's hand went up. "I want to tell other students not to give up if they are being bullied and to talk to parents and teachers and their principal and anyone else, but don't ever give up!" Then she stood up and broke into her rap, with her two backup singers supporting her. We were all getting excited about the show.

At our last rehearsal, Wendy told me she wanted to dedicate the rap song to her mother. "I want to thank her for all she did for me." On the afternoon of the show, the group of student actors and their ENACT coaches stood backstage holding hands in a silent prayer. They had formed a special kind of family, filling an essential need for many students.

The lights went up, and they took their places on the stage, looking proud and confident. Stepping out under the lights, witnessed by a supportive audience, these students had transformed from the roles of the "Dropout" to the roles of "Empowered Messengers." Their transformation was witnessed under shining lights for all to see, changing the perceptions of everyone in that audience.

Wendy's mother sat in the auditorium's front row, beaming as her daughter performed the closing rap number under a spotlight, with the two backup singers behind her. A confident young lady stood transformed, finally revealing the powerful person she had hidden for so long. While each group member had shed the role of the Dropout, Wendy had also shed the role of The Victim. Each group member was now embracing their authentic, empowered self through the role of the "Performer."

When the lights dimmed and the spotlight appeared around her, Wendy looked down at her mother in the audience and said, "Thank you, Mom, for always being there for me. You were my greatest support." The lights went down, and the curtain closed. Her mom, joined by the entire audience, was moved to tears, on their feet, clapping and cheering.

Author's Notes

- Wendy transformed from the role of Victim to the role of Performer. Through the framework of theater, she turned her traumatic experience and talents into a message about bullying that could help others. Her negative self-concept was transformed into a positive one, witnessed by a supportive community.
- Students in the class let go of negative self-concepts, in the role of The Dropout, taking on positive ones, in the role of The Empowered Performer, as witnessed by an audience.
- The performance acted as a vehicle to mobilize around the issue of cyberbullying plaguing youth around the country. These youth shared a collective voice, a powerful tool for healing.
- Being witnessed on a stage under the lights is a magical way to empower even the most self-conscious youth to rise to the occasion.

The aftermath of trauma leaves a lot of collateral damage. But there is hope. As the field of trauma continues to develop, growing research and new approaches to healing trauma are spreading through school systems and other youth-serving organizations. There is a movement toward trauma-informed classrooms. We are beginning to understand how intense stress and fear disrupt the nervous system and how they can be reversed with compassionate care. Frameworks like SEL (social and emotional learning) help youth recognize and manage feelings. New appreciation for the arts, such as drawing, music, and dance, are being studied as sound approaches and creative arts practices are finally integrated into many youth-serving programs.

ENACT has worked successfully with hundreds of thousands of teens in classrooms and youth settings in New York City and across the country, where more traditional therapeutic methods may not have reached them. The ENACT Method is designed for youth to be truly seen for who they are, allowing them to relinquish their protective roles, resulting in remarkable breakthroughs.

Notes

1 Blaustein, *Treating Traumatic Stress in Children and Adolescents*, 27.
2 Blaustein, *Treating Traumatic Stress in Children and Adolescents*, 29.
3 Levine, *Waking the Tiger*, 169.
4 Ogdon, *Trauma and the Body*, 92.
5 Ogdon, *Trauma and the Body*, 96.

6 Blaustein, *Treating Traumatic Stress in Children and Adolescents*, 30.
7 van der Kolk, *The Body Keeps the Score*, 6.
8 Mate, *The Myth of Normal.*
9 Mate, *The Myth of Normal.*
10 Mate, *The Myth of Normal*, 225.
11 National Center for Education Statistics, The Condition of Education 2024, Chapter 2. Accessed July 27, 2025 at: https://nces.ed.gov/programs/coe/indicator/a10/bullying-electronic-bullying#:~:text=In%202019%2C%20about%2022%20percent,during%20the%20previous%2012%20months.
12 Mate, *The Myth of Normal*, 185. [Gabor Mate – quoting Gordon Neufeld]
13 Pipher, *Reviving Ophelia*, 158.
14 Journal of American Academy of Child and Adolescent Psychiatry in journal 10, updated 2023. https://www.aacap.org/AACAP/Families_and_Youth/Facts_for_Families/FFF-Guide/Teen-Suicide-010.aspx

Chapter 4

False Selves/Roles

"Finish lunch and finish it now!" a full-bodied security guard hollered. "You have three minutes. So, eat!"

The teenagers receiving this command to scarf down their hospital food had been tagged as having "behavioral problems" and placed in this school unit, an educational institution based in a hospital designed for students who cannot attend traditional schools due to severe emotional and behavioral challenges. Depending on their progress, these students could be there anywhere from a semester to several years. They tended to be violent to themselves and others and were on constant watch. They came in on an outpatient basis, meaning that each day after school they went home, usually to foster homes or very troubled families.

The small cafeteria was our workplace. Several hospital staff members floated in and out. Confident with 12 years of experience working with kids who had behavior problems, I had brought a trusted and skilled sidekick-partner, Marco, a strong, sensitive Latinx actor who offered an excellent role model for many of the youth. Still, this situation would be a challenge.

I first worked to bring out the confidence and creativity in Lucy, an adolescent tagged by her teacher as "a suicide case." I was also told that she wanted to be an actress. But my attention shifted because of James, a 16-year-old tagged as having an "irresolvable behavioral problem."

At least once a day, James would threaten Lucy, saying, "Don't look at me again, or I'll kill you." Lucy would retreat deeper into her chair.

DOI: 10.4324/9781003415022-6

"Don't look at me, or I'll kill you." "Get out of my face." "Leave me alone." Comments like these are defenses that teens often use to prevent their unwanted emotions from emerging. James created the role of "Bully" to compensate for his poor self-concept and to avoid his painful feelings of shame. Misunderstood defenses are common for teens who get labeled as "troubled" or tagged with "behavior problems." But despite their appearance, defenses are not "bad behavior"; they are forms of emotional survival. Youth with unhealed trauma are like proud warriors who use their defense mechanisms as weapons to shield them from harm and fight off anyone or anything that poses a threat, real or imagined.

When confronted with these aggressive attitudes, people retreat because they feel intimidated. For now, these adolescents have won the battle but lost the war because, in the long run, they have not met their underlying needs or addressed the fear beneath the defense.

Roles as Accommodations

Teens create roles as accommodations. They compensate for the environments where they grew up and where they live currently. They anticipate danger and mobilize defenses.

I understood this when The New York City Council funded the ENACT Dropout Prevention Program in the early 2000s to improve school attendance in neighborhoods with high levels of poverty and crime. During our weekly group discussions, I came to know and care about our students. When we asked the kids with long-term absences why they had missed so many days, they revealed that they felt their home environments and neighborhoods were so unsafe that just getting up to go to school was a significant challenge. They told us that they were sometimes too depressed to get out of bed or they struggled with so much anxiety they couldn't get to sleep the night before. They made accommodations for their situations with humor, bravery, and determination. They developed creative coping skills by playing roles, presenting themselves as fearless and invulnerable, covering up their underlying feelings of helplessness and fear. Their peers accepted their roles, but teachers and other adults perceived them as oppositional or defiant.

These teens likely had experienced developmental trauma and, as accommodations for upsetting, vulnerable emotions, portrayed the opposite, untouchable versions of themselves. Underneath, they were scared and wounded, and they knew it. They were scarred by neglect and or abuse, felt shame, and often blamed themselves for their situations. They deserved a chance to fulfill their potential but were stuck in their roles. If offered help, they usually turned it down out of fear or pride.

Enter ENACT is a therapeutic theater program that worked directly with students in their classrooms using nontraditional, fun, and engaging methods to help them address their issues. The students were willing and interested in participating in the program and reported that they enjoyed it and learned important things about themselves. ENACT was often called into schools for behavioral interventions because of its positive effects on behavior change. Evidence-based evaluations demonstrated this. Behavior change has the best and most lasting results when working with underlying issues that cause the behavior.

Internalizing Negative Labels and Reinforcing Roles[1]

Teachers and others who work with youth in school classrooms and observe them in halls and cafeterias may label those who habitually play roles. Without the proper tools or understanding, it is easier to brand them as having "behavior problems" or as "troubled," "acting out," or "bad" than it is to get to the source of the problem. Labels reinforce the behavior and the youth's negative self-concept. The labels become internalized and strengthen their roles. I recall when I worked in a classroom with students labeled as "acting out," and a student introduced the group to me. "We are the Bad Ones, right?" they asked, as if wanting confirmation of the given label.

If a student's behavior is caused by trauma and an adult punishes them for having "bad behavior," the negative label gets internalized and becomes their adopted role. For years, I saw students in public schools play the same roles repeatedly. The "acting-out" role was popular.

The "shut-down" role was another. The Class Clown had many versions as well. Sometimes, it was difficult to differentiate the student from their role because it was so habitual for them to play it that it became intertwined with their personalities.

Stuck in a Role

Working with students in New York City classrooms for more than three decades, I observed patterns in their behaviors. I saw how students with developmental trauma lived inside of self-created roles with protective armor (defensive responses). Their postures, facial expressions, and tone of voice became exaggerated whenever they felt insecure or afraid of danger. Unfortunately, this was most of the time. As explained earlier, these feelings likely started early in their lives. Their defenses were their survival mechanisms, shielding them from feeling vulnerable. By helping them to become conscious of the defended parts of themselves, we were able to help many of these students to release their long-held "stuck" emotions and find safe avenues for expression. This also helped them discover new parts of themselves and improve their self-concept.

It has been my experience that if a role is excessively played out, it becomes chronic. Performed repeatedly, the body holds postures and attitudes as if imprinted in the body. The role becomes a mold that is difficult to break out of. The creator gets **stuck in a role.**

In her sensory motor work, Pat Ogden explains how the structure of a body posture is stored in the individual muscle patterns, remaining rigid and inflexible. Similar to the way trauma lodges in the body, roles, too, can get stuck in the body, constricting the possibility of another more expansive expression. ENACT's theater games allowed youth to rediscover play, a spontaneous experience that expanded their ability for flexibility and joy.

Role Types

Inspired by Robert Landy's groundbreaking work on role theory,[2] I have observed recurrent adolescent role types over many years of working with teens. A compilation of this sort can help teachers, parents, and adults view adolescent behavior with an understanding of youth's adaptive mechanisms. Of course, people are not static beings; personalities change, and role types are not set in stone. I also know that listing types, stereotypes, or labels can feel elemental. However, when viewed through a theatrical lens, their creativity can be appreciated. ENACT's role-play method, portraying typical observable roles seen in the classroom, helped our actors and teaching artists deliver our method successfully in hundreds of classrooms to thousands of students across New York City. With an understanding of role adaptations, adults can find new ways to work with youth and avoid getting caught in the drama.

Below is a chart of common adolescent role types depicting characters with strong defenses used to block difficult emotions. Please note this is only a partial list and is viewed through our lens in a Western culture. These roles may mean something very different in different cultures.

Adolescent Roles

1	The Class Clown	15	The Hyper One
2	The Bully	16	The Apathetic One
3	The Victim	17	The Spacy One
4	The Defiant One	18	The Resistant One
5	The Child	19	The Aggressor
6	The Motherless Child	20	The Shut-Down One
7	The Isolated One	21	The Liar
8	The Tough One	22	The Loser
9	The Blamer	23	The Operator
10	The Voiceless One	24	The Gangster
11	The Avoidant One	25	The Leader
12	The Bad One	26	The Follower
13	The Survivor	27	The Troublemaker
14	The Seducer	28	The Belligerent One

Protective Roles as Shields against Vulnerability

The core of the ENACT role-play method is working creatively with youth defensive responses in a safe, indirect way, using professional actors to foster engagement and self-reflection. The ENACT role-play process allows teens to become conscious observers of their protective armor and, over time, recover lost parts of themselves to reclaim their authentic selves.

Working with teens to incorporate their defensive responses into the process of change can be challenging for practitioners who use traditional forms of therapy. A mind-body approach is likely to be more effective. Youth with unhealed trauma have layered defenses that need to be unpeeled one at a time to reinstate more flexible functioning. This must be done at their readiness level, with them in the driver's seat.

Trauma cuts off a sense of control, and teens depend on their defenses as a way to maintain that control. Therefore, trying to remove defenses too quickly will backfire.

Using actors to mirror participants' defenses allows teens a safe way to self-reflect by observing others having a parallel experience. Only when students acknowledge their defenses and become consciously aware of them can they work on a process of change.

Using the term "a true self" or "an authentic self," I refer to behavior connected to one's emotions and body without significant defenses. When we "play a role" or "embody a false self," we separate ourselves from our authenticity. Youth who suffer from unhealed trauma often push troublesome emotions out of conscious awareness. They fear these feelings will be overwhelming and unmanageable, so they mask and push them away. But the feelings do not disappear; they are stored in the body, held in muscular patterns and postures. We see this in the roles the students play. Defenses aim to protect buried feelings from emerging, so as practitioners, we need to be mindful to respect them and to use indirect methods to address them.

One day, while doing a scene for a class, I felt I needed to go deeper with the process. I discovered a safe way to work with defenses by creating a portal to self-awareness: *the inner monologue.* I stopped a role-play at the point of high conflict and asked our seasoned actor to stop the action and do an inner monologue voicing their character's fears and insecurity: *I'm afraid if I don't act tough, he will see that I am weak, and I don't know what could happen. I have enough problems at home; I don't need any more from him, too.* The inner monologue expressed for the students what they could not express themselves. It "let the cat out of the bag."

The postures and facial expressions of the students observing the monologue told me that an unspoken connection had been made. They were nodding their heads as if they understood, and I knew we had hit a sweet spot because they also exhibited these protective behaviors.

Through quiet recognition, an opening was made for personal reflection, and the students were ready to go further in a deepening process. ENACT's "outside, inside" method was born, which became a signature tool of our work. Working to unwind defenses by mirroring external behavior and externalizing internal feelings became the key to reaching highly defended youth and engaging them in conscious transformation.

The goal of the ENACT Method is to help teens become self-aware as they move past the barriers of a false self, portrayed in roles, and connect back to their true selves, allowing for emotional integration and conscious transformation.

Roles can only be played in social contexts; interaction with others is needed to express them. Peer groups are especially important to teens. For many young people, peers become increasingly valuable when they forge identities separate from their families. Unfortunately, to be accepted by a peer group, teens often give up their authentic thoughts and feelings, making them more vulnerable to peer pressure. They feel they must keep up their false self/role to be a valuable group member and can dress, act, and participate in self-destructive behaviors to gain peer approval. Roles are accommodations for parts of the self that are not "good enough" or considered acceptable. Sometimes, they are developed to compensate for negative self-beliefs from adverse attachment experiences.

Creating a role is sometimes in response to peer pressure. But there are other reasons people play roles. Actors perform roles to entertain and to relate emotional material to an audience. The safe distance of theater allows the audience to experience empathy that may result in cathartic reactions such as laughter or tears. This is why we often hear thunderous applause when an audience is moved to tears by a performance.

Like actors, teens create roles and act out real-life dramas through interpersonal relationships. But their show is not performed in a theater, and they don't receive applause.

They play their role all day, every day, on the stage of life, in schools, neighborhoods, and sometimes in their homes. They write their scripts and design behavioral costumes that match the essence of the role through attitudes, facial expressions, and gestures.

Teens are generally drawn to high drama and conflict; it reflects their inner turbulence. Teens who have experienced trauma understand the intense anxiety, confusion, and pain portrayed in the dramatic characters they see on television and in movies. Many teens like to perform the ENACT scenarios because it is a safe way to express themselves. It is also freeing.

Teens who have experienced trauma may greatly benefit from role-play because trauma causes constriction of thoughts and feelings. Role-play allows for freedom of expression; individuals can find and express their voices within the safe context of theater. It can help them reconnect to their lost parts, find authenticity, and express the unspoken.

The ENACT Method uses the technique of theatrical distancing: representing an emotion or situation with emotional honesty but with just enough of a difference to ensure the safety needed for teens to connect to themselves and others. Teens who have experienced trauma often have difficulty with relationships, particularly if they have experienced attachment trauma. Role-play is perfect for them to practice interacting and verbalizing their thoughts and feelings. Since trauma is stored in the body, experiential activities like role-playing allow for an embodied experience with spontaneous expression and action. Role-playing encourages risk-taking and provides a platform for meaning-making.

In the ENACT work, teens rehearse real-life situations and work through issues and challenges relevant to their lives. Witnessed by an audience of supportive peers, role-playing allows youth to work through challenges and know they are not alone.

The ENACT role-play method is designed for a process of change, as teens try on new roles and let go of others. It is a rehearsal for life.

The ENACT Method draws even the most resistant youth into a process of self-reflection and discovery through the signature role-play method. This carefully constructed process offers opportunities for reflection for highly defended youth who might not otherwise be reached.

In classrooms throughout New York City, thousands of students, many of whom sometimes seemed almost impossible to reach, would participate in the role-play method, resulting in externalizing thoughts and feelings and finding new meaning in their lives.

The Downside to Relinquishing a Role

In some cases of undergoing transformation, there is a danger. This is especially true for youth who live in unsafe environments. A student once told me, "If I express my real emotions on the street in my neighborhood, I could get jumped. I need to act cool."

He was right! We needed to appreciate the context in which our youth lived, which, for many, were neighborhoods with high rates of poverty and crime. Their environment often dictated their roles, and they needed highly defended behavior to protect themselves. While our aim was to help them manage and transform their behavior, responses like hypervigilance or fight-flight responses might have saved them on the street. It would have been unjust for us, and dangerous for them, to ignore the fact that protective behavior was often needed to shield them from genuine threats. In his book *Introduction to Internal Family Systems*, Dr. Richard Schwartz describes his work in urban schools, explaining that he understood that some students could not afford to "drop their protective wall of defiance and bravado in their neighborhoods because they were at risk of being attacked if they were vulnerable."[3]

Helping youth become conscious of their roles and defenses by shining a light on their authentic selves allows them to make conscious choices about how and when to use their role. But our work does not change the structural conditions that exist for many of these teens, including poverty and racism. I am grateful to social advocates who are fighting for change.

Role Functions

The ENACT role-play method employs two primary role categories: **Compensatory and Protective.**

The Compensatory Role is a mostly conscious coping mechanism to accommodate for an individual's poor self-concept. An individual will superimpose a new "self" to replace the old to gain acceptance in social situations. In Robert Landy's pioneering book, *Drama Therapy, Persona, and Performance*, he explains that role-choosing suggests a conscious decision on the person's part to take on the desired qualities of someone they admire. He states that "role...is very much at the center of the personality."[4] We often see compensatory roles played in youth demonstrated through how they dress and relate to one another with exaggerated attitudes and gestures. These roles are designed to gain approval from others. But they are also designed for self-acceptance.

Unlike the compensatory role, **the Protective Role** is unconscious. Through highly protective defenses, this role prevents difficult emotions and memories from emerging. We can see these defenses in the physicality of youth with rigid postural body armor, resistant behavior toward others, extreme attitudes, and guarded gestures.

The ENACT role-play method fully explores teens' protective defenses. Their defenses dictate their interaction in the scene, allowing them to feel a sense of control, which is essential for youth with trauma who may feel powerless. Teens can experience a sense of power when they play a character in a scene with the same defenses they use daily. They know how to portray characters who express behaviors like avoidance, denial, and aggression.

Some teens, especially those with a history of trauma, can become easily activated in role-play since role-plays are unscripted and spontaneous. From time to time, adolescents may get so immersed in the scenario that they lose control. In this case, they need an anchor to help them emotionally regulate. It is the function of ENACT coaches to stand behind the student actors, assisting them in keeping their boundaries and controlling their behavior when needed. The ENACT director also initiates directives like "freeze" and "focus" and may stop a scene if a student becomes too activated or uncontrolled. Role-play can be a great way to allow youth to practice self-regulation skills. It is also a means of assessment, as we can observe the adolescents' positive and negative self-beliefs through the roles they choose to play.

The Protective Role and Developmental Trauma

The ENACT Method calls for actors to take on a version of the protective roles teens inhabit. In doing so, they demonstrate teens' strong defenses of denial, resistance, and aggression as coping mechanisms in conflict scenes portraying interactions with peers and adults. The use of the protective roles has proven extremely effective in reaching teens with extreme resistance.

A typical ENACT classroom scene involves a conflict between a teacher and a highly reactive student, like the one that begins the Introduction to this book. The teacher's lesson is interrupted when Troy, a boisterous student, comes barreling into the classroom, talking to other students and ignoring the teacher's instructions for him to settle down.

"Leave me alone!" he says. "You are interrupting my class!" she responds. Embodying the protective role to mirror the defenses of individuals in the group, the actor portrays the student's defense of apathy, acting as if he doesn't care. As the confrontation heightens, he becomes defiant. "Leave me alone," he yells, "you always pick on me!"

_____

As the students watch the scene, they become fully engaged because it resonates with them. They see themselves in the role of the character. They understand the defenses because they have the same.

_____

When Troy does an inner monologue, revealing his core emotion of hopelessness because he believes he will not pass the class, several students empathize and become even more connected.

This indirect approach is a safe initial step toward introspection and conscious transformation. This is beneficial for youth with developmental trauma, who are often unable to access and address the trauma of neglect and abuse caused by early caregivers because it has been pushed out of their conscious awareness.

Protective roles serve a purpose. As drama therapist Renée Emunah explains, "the theatrical role of a character, like a mask, is protective and liberating, enabling the expression of what lies beneath our real-life roles."[5] However, taking on these roles can also prevent youth from connecting to their authentic selves, the part of them that is creative, spontaneous, and alive. By reuniting with their true selves *and* integrating their emotions, thoughts, and perceptions, they have the opportunity for healing.

A student I encountered, named John, was like Troy in the ENACT scenario above. John was always late for class, was disruptive when he arrived, and would ignore the teacher's demands for better behavior, even when the teacher threatened to fail him. Nonetheless, John would keep acting like he didn't care. He was playing the role of The Belligerent One. Upon further investigation, we found out that John was in the process of being moved into a foster care system. Underneath his role, John felt incredibly vulnerable. He worked so hard to hide his feelings that he was stuck in a role and unwilling to ask for help.

Underlying Needs

Taking on particular roles often reflects the unconscious need for acceptance, validation, and respect, core to human growth and development. Protective roles played by youth, such as The Defiant One, portray behaviors that aim to meet these needs. Despite the deep desire for connection and acceptance, they often protect themselves from the very thing they're seeking. A student described with "difficult behavior" is not purposely being difficult. They are trying to gain attention and validation, likely missing from their upbringing, from peers and adults. If not positive attention, then negative attention will suffice.

Do not be fooled. An adolescent's role is often used as a cover to disguise their emotions to "save face."

Teens will hide undesirable feelings like shame and fear beneath the guise of a defensive mask and will create roles that portray the opposite of how they feel.

These are coping mechanisms and accommodations for poor self-concept. An example of a role opposite would be the adolescent who feels depressed and portrays the role of The Class Clown, exhibiting goofy behavior, laughing, and cracking jokes. Underneath the behavior, they are sad and lonely. Another example would be a student suffering from isolation but compensating by playing the role of an effervescent "social butterfly."

Role Reinforcement

Role reinforcement is important to youth. They are seeking attention. Their peers' approval, through laughter or imitation, reinforces their role. However, a failed attempt at attention can backfire and invoke negative attention from peers and adults. Teens who have early attachment wounds and push away a significant adult, such as a teacher, may confront a painful reminder of past experiences with caregivers. The current rupture unconsciously or consciously reminds them of early neglectful or abusive relationships and can feel terrible.

Over the years, I often saw students playing roles like The Class Clown or The Aggressor, which would provoke a teacher or other adult to respond by calling them out for their behavior and shaming them in front of their peers. In the case history introduced at the start of this chapter, James was disciplined for being a bully, but unfortunately, the root cause of his behavior went unaddressed. The accusation induced feelings of humiliation and did not lead him to change his role but only reinforced it.

Role as a Defense against Shame

Shame has been described as "the feeling of being bad, unworthy of being alive."[6] It activates feelings of low self-esteem, anger, and depression.

Adolescents are known to feel shame more acutely than adults, and may protect themselves against these feelings by creating roles that include resistant or oppositional behavior. For example, a student may react angrily if they feel put on the spot by a well-meaning teacher who asks them to come up to the blackboard to answer a question. They may get triggered by the suggestion, especially if they are unsure of the answer, and to avoid shame, they jump into retaliatory behavior by throwing down a book, yelling, or stomping out of the classroom.

Chronic feelings of shame can be dangerous to a vulnerable youth; it can lead to feelings of self-hatred. Self-destructive behaviors can turn into violence, self-harm, or even suicide. Adults who work with teens must be on the lookout for shame responses in their youth. They must be sensitive to shame's harmful effects and become the teen's best allies. Adults can help youth feel protected from the unwanted impacts of shame by immediately spotting and stopping shaming by their peers when they see it. They can try to counterbalance the effects of shame by normalizing the feeling and reinforcing the youth's strengths, talents, and positive qualities. Positive insights and beliefs can be instilled and reinforced by continually letting the youth know they are fine as they are, they are safe, and they are worthy.

Role as a Form of Dissociation

Dissociation is a clear indication of trauma. We say that someone is *dissociated* when they severely distance themselves from their feelings to avoid emotional pain. It could be argued that the unconscious creation of a role is a form of the dissociative process because it separates the individual from the authentic self and creates a stand-in personality to supersede it. An individual with dissociative symptoms can seem "zoned out" and, when asked how they feel, may genuinely not know because they have emotionally left their bodies. Uninformed teachers or other adults may yell at them, demanding that they pay attention, but it is almost impossible for individuals in this state. While it may look as if they are present, they are not. Their role may be standing in for them. An adolescent with dissociation may feel numb, and their role gives them something to connect to.

An adult in a relationship with a dissociated youth may feel frustrated or take it personally when the youth does not connect with them. But teens who do this are disconnected from themselves. If dissociation occurs, grounding techniques like art and movement and embodied activities like role-play offer a safe, indirect container to help youth reconnect to themselves. Dissociation denies individuals the opportunity to connect to their true thoughts and feelings. A role may temporarily replace them, but the outcome is the same. Their authentic self is far, far away. The goal of working with anyone with dissociation is to help them find their way back to a safe, embodied self.

To continue our focus on role, we return to the story of James, started at the beginning of this chapter, who had taken on the role of The Bully. James was snapping at his classmate with violent threats.

At first, I tried to ignore James' behavior. Mistake! Frustrated by the end of the week, I had to do something. This behavior was what I was supposed to "manage."

James often hid his face, and I finally realized it was because it was covered in acne. I noticed he looked away whenever I looked at him, as if trying to disappear. There was something he was hiding. Something he was ashamed of. "That's it!" I thought. The poor guy, I realized, not only had to bear adolescence's unfairness in a hospital unit, he had to do so with a face that shamed him. He defended against this feeling by playing the role of The Bully.

I quickly devised a scenario that would protect him against further shame, hoping that he would connect to the same core feeling the character was experiencing in a parallel scene. I asked Marco to play a scene with me involving two co-workers, one of whom had burns on his hands.

Playing this part, Marco would say, "Please don't look at my hands," hiding them behind his back. Without my antagonizing him, his threats grew more hostile until he threatened my life. "If you look at me one more time, I'll kill you!" he finally yelled. I froze in character, and the scene ended.

James's hand was the first to shoot up when we asked the students what was happening in the scene. "The character feels mad, and he's a bully," he said. "That's why he threatened you." At that moment, his voice softened, as did his eyes. His whole body melted into his chair. Other students volunteered ideas as well.

Rather than push James beyond his comfort zone or risk causing him further feelings of shame, we returned to the magic of drama. We recruited different students to play out possible endings to the scene. James was the first to volunteer as the hostile co-worker, saying, "Look, I burned my hands, and I am embarrassed. Okay? So, please stop drawing attention to it. If you look at them, everyone will look." In another possible ending, Lucy played the role of the threatened co-worker and said, "I feel bad about how I look sometimes, too. So, don't feel bad. Your hands look better than you might think they do."

We had a breakthrough! Both students identified feelings of shame. We explained shame, named it, demystified it, and normalized it. Cultivating awareness and speaking about the unspoken in a nonjudgmental way cuts to the root cause of the behavior. I saw many heads nodding as if they all understood the issue, which was a deep feeling of shame. But rather than speaking to James afterward, I ran up to Lucy, asking her if she understood why James threatened her daily. Her usual shutdown body posture opened up, and she said, "Yeah. He is embarrassed. It's not me!" She beamed.

Author's Notes

- We disregarded the student's labels and nudged transformation. Teens are sensitive to labels. "Unreachable case" (Lucy) and "irresolvable behavioral problem" (James) are extreme examples. It turns out the "unreachable case" wanted to become an actress, while the "behavioral problem" wanted what we all want—respect.
- James was likely bullied himself, and possibly in his own home. We identified the underlying core emotion—shame—and found a way to externalize it for the group through a distanced role-play.
- Students identified and named the emotion.
- We encouraged self-awareness by helping to name and demystify the feeling.

The breakthrough experienced by James was unforgettable. Through my work with ENACT, I have observed many such breakthroughs and transformations. As discussed above, the power of role-play offers individuals the safety and freedom to find and express their voice. They can experiment with new ways of communicating and practice interacting with others.

To end this chapter, I add another remarkable story, this one about a young woman I will call Robin, who stopped speaking after she was raped by her boyfriend. Robin found her voice again in an ENACT role-play.[7] Because Robin became selectively mute to deal with this trauma, I call her role, and this case history, The Silenced One.

Twelve teenage girls were placed in a specialized hospital school because of their risky behaviors. Some had self-harming behaviors, others were suicidal—several had experienced severe neglect, abuse, and trauma. Robin was described to me as being selectively mute and "almost catatonic" by her social worker, who reported that she could only communicate through puppets with her psychiatrist. I was told that Robin had been raped by her new boyfriend and hadn't spoken a word for the months following.

When we begin working with a new group of students, we invite the participants to join us, standing up in the circle. But reading the girls' guarded emotional states, my partner and I assumed the group preferred to stay in the safety of their chairs, so we greeted them individually. When I approached Robin each day, she looked away as if she was trying to disappear. She slumped more deeply into her chair.

Aware that several of the girls had experienced abuse in their homes or their relationships, we wanted to ensure that they felt safe, protected, and respected in our space. Group unison games where we all did actions at the same time allowed everyone to work together and no one to stand out. As the games progressed, the students became more spontaneous and playful. A few more students joined the circle each day. Robin watched from her chair with growing interest every day.

One day, when I greeted her, Robin raised her head and smiled at me for the first time. I smiled back, and a connection was made between us. She seemed more approachable each day but wasn't ready to join the circle. Honoring her boundaries, we began with unison games from their chairs, where she participated nonverbally. One day, we invited all the students to join the circle. Robin must have felt safe enough to participate because she got up from her chair and joined the circle. As each day progressed, Robin would mouth her words and eventually whisper them. She was beginning to open up.

The group was bonding through the theater games as Robin experimented with her voice, sometimes moving her mouth without words, other times speaking softly. Once the group members seemed comfortable, I asked them what issues they wanted to work on. "Boy-friends," several of them voiced. This was our opportunity to broach the topic of relationship abuse, but carefully. A parallel scene would allow them the emotional distance needed to address the issue.

The scene revolves around Jessie, the girlfriend, and Jerry, an abusive boyfriend. It opens with Jessie and Jerry speaking on the phone about a party he insists on attending that night. He asks Jessie to join him, but she declines, saying she doesn't feel well. He becomes angry and begins with tactics to pressure her. The more she explains that she isn't up to it and has homework, the more angry and increasingly threatening Jerry becomes.

"You are supposed to be my girlfriend," he begins shouting, "and girlfriends don't leave their guys to go to parties alone! You are hurting me," he says dramatically, "and you will regret it!" He tells her he plans to come to her house and pull her by her hair if she is not ready. The scene ends when the doorbell rings, and Jessie stands frozen with the phone in her hand. An inner monologue expresses her fear and distress.

Following the scene, the youth processed the characters' feelings, bridging them to connect to their own thoughts and feelings. When we asked them for potential solutions, the group was united in find-ing solutions to help Jessie stand up for herself. Robin watched and listened intently.

"Does anyone want to come up here and try out some of these possible solutions?" I asked. "I want to play the boyfriend," a student said. Then, unexpectedly, from the back of the room, Robin declared, "I want to play the girlfriend." We confirmed her decision, worried she could get retraumatized, but she con-fidently walked up to the stage. I stood behind her in case she needed me to ensure her safety.

Robin and her classmate replayed the scene together. At the final dramatic moment, when the doorbell rang, Robin stepped out of character, turned to her classmates, and said confidently, "Don't ever let anyone talk to you that way, and don't ever let anyone threaten you. Never let anyone hit you!" she declared in an em-powered voice no one had heard from her before. This was the first time they had heard her speak out. The room was silent and then broke into thunderous applause. Trauma had robbed Robin of her voice, and through the role-play, she had found it again.

Robin stood on the stage that day, grounded, fully embodied, and looking different. She was now powerful and brave. We had the honor of watching Robin transform from a victim to a courageous survivor. She proudly took a bow. Her classmates cheered again, "Yay, Robin!"

When the session ended, the social worker told me that she had never heard Robin utter a word. "I can't believe what I have just witnessed," she said. "I am going to tell her therapist immediately!"

On our last day of class, an awards ceremony was held. My teaching partner played the master of ceremonies. She handed each student an award acknowledging their progress and their strengths. Robin received her certificate and read it aloud, "To Robin, who found her voice." She took a bow. The class cheered.

Author's Notes

This was a stunning case with a quick breakthrough. The timing was right, and all the elements came together.

- We worked developmentally with Robin, starting with nonverbal exercises, meeting her where she was, and building from there.
- The topic of abuse was indirectly addressed through a carefully designed scene with the proper distance. The scene focused on a relationship instead of abuse. Focusing on the character's relationships instead of the issue is a good rule of thumb because it provides more distance.
- The group acted as a supportive container and a witness to Robin's transformation.
- Robin found a platform to discover and express voice through the magic of theater.
- Success was celebrated with a written certificate of accomplishment. Celebrating success is an excellent way for individuals to have evidence of accomplishment and growth.

Notes

1 ENACT program evaluation Rob Horowitz, New York Center for Arts Education Research (2011).
2 Landy, *Persona and Performance*.
3 Schwartz, *Introduction to Internal Family Systems*, 77.
4 Landy, *Persona and Performance*, 38.
5 Emunah, *Acting for Real*, 7.
6 Fisher, *Neurofeedback in the Treatment of Developmental Trauma*, 24.
7 Feldman, *Current Approaches in Drama Therapy*, 305.

Chapter 5

Intersections of Theater and Therapy

Whenever I work with any group, I begin collecting impressions without labeling or judging what I see, which is a first step—maybe even the key—to connecting.

This assignment was not a typical one for ENACT; we were working with a group of young children with autism. In this school setting, about a dozen eight- and nine-year-olds swirled around like wound-up toy boats let loose in a pool. One girl spun in circles like a small Sufi dancer. Several kids rocked repetitively back and forth. A boy with his arms extended zoomed like a plane in and out of the other kids' space. Others played with colored blocks next to each other, but they did not play together. There was a boy wearing a crash helmet, another one wearing an oversized sweatshirt and too-long pants dirty at the hems from being stepped on. What struck me was that although the room was filled with movement and inarticulate groans and other sounds, nobody in that room was interacting with anyone else. Each child was on his or her own planet.

While part of my mind was assessing what I sensed—trying to evaluate the children's motor skills, for instance—the next step for me was tuning in to what I felt, making space for the beginnings of empathy. I tried to connect one-on-one with several of the children, giving them a warm smile and a touch on their small hands, but they didn't react; they seemed more interested in the feeling of the objects they were holding or in the repetitive motions of their own arms.

When I opened myself to these children, trying to feel what they felt, in a flash, it came to me—isolated! I needed to find a symbol or character that felt the same way, that would speak to them without actually speaking, something that could express for

DOI: 10.4324/9781003415022-7

them what they couldn't express. What was the symbol or character we needed here? The answer came to me loud and clear: a lonely Moon Man isolated on his own planet.

Empathetically attuned to the children, I became fully present, allowing myself to let go and trust my intuition. When I felt the isolation of these students, it allowed impressions to emerge. That's when the metaphor of an isolated Moon Man appeared.

The shared goal of therapy and theater has always been to inspire individuals to gain self-awareness. In both disciplines, a technique for achieving this (as illustrated above) is **empathetic attunement.** The ENACT drama therapy method incorporates professional actors into the process who, through empathetic attunement, can observe participants and reflect back their impressions using various theater/drama techniques, such as theater games and role-play. **Attunement, empathetic attunement**, and **embodied attunement** are all important concepts that will be covered in more detail later in this chapter. At the end of this chapter, you can read the story of how the Moon Man came to life for these children, and the magical transformation that came about because of empathetic attunement.

Guiding Theater Concepts

The ENACT method is rooted in theater and therapy. It is a drama therapy method that uses actors and specific applications of theater games, improvisation, and role-play to help youth achieve psychological growth and change.

The ENACT method uses theater applications such as theater games, improvisation, and role-play to achieve personal growth and transformation. These theatrical applications are adjusted to meet therapeutic goals. Below is a discussion of traditional theater methods and how ENACT adapts them for therapeutic change.

Improvisation

Improvisation is a form of acting that takes place right in the moment. It is spontaneous and playful, allowing individuals to open up to their creativity. Improvisation also fosters trust because you must rely on others to move a scene forward. There is generally no planning, set script, or specific plot; it is a fun, freeing, theatrical experience, but works within specific guidelines, such as agreeing with the other player and avoiding the word "no," to keep the action going.

You do not need to be an actor to use the basic skills of improvisation, such as agreeing with your scene partner in order to keep the dialogue going. Improvisation is often taught in business to help leaders connect their teams, and salespeople to connect with their clients. In fact, it has also helped FBI agents negotiate in hostage situations. Improvisation is a powerful tool that is relevant to theater and other communication fields.

ENACT Application of Improvisation

ENACT uses a structured form of improvisation. The roles are assigned. The plot is minimally planned, and the role-play has particular start and stop points for audience reflection and participation. Improvisations are used for therapeutic purposes and to teach social and emotional skills.

Role-Play

Role-play is usually performed in a group setting in which characters spontaneously interact with each other. Often, there are objectives and the roles are portrayed in a predetermined time and place. Like improvisation, role-play uses acting to imitate the behavior of someone different from themselves. Like improvisation, role-play is used in many arenas beyond acting classes. It can help teach communication skills in the workplace, business settings, and schools. It is a perfect tool for learning life skills, as participants can rehearse for real-life situations.

ENACT Application of Role-Play

Within a preplanned scene, two characters portray a scene in a particular context relatable to the audience. The scene builds up to an unresolved conflict that becomes increasingly heightened until the characters stop the action and deliver monologues revealing their inner thoughts and feelings. The aim is to have the participants understand behavior and the underlying emotions that drive it as a first step toward more positive and productive social interactions.

Character/Role

In performance, an actor assumes the role of a fictional character in a play to bring a story to life. They communicate ideas and feelings through consciously created personas. Characters are played in theater, film, television, and online. They are also portrayed in video games, with avatars representing the players.

ENACT Application of Character/Role

The ENACT Method uses actors to portray roles that reflect the underlying needs of youth, which are externalized through the behavior of the role. The aim is to build trust by having participants empathize with the characters in a scene to create a feeling of connectedness and prepare them for the next stages of the work. Similarly, scenes are created that are relevant to the lives of the participants. ENACT uses two kinds of roles to reach different goals: the compensatory role and the protective role.

- **The Compensatory Role**: This role is consciously designed as a false self, created to imitate an admired figure to gain social acceptance. In an ENACT session, this role is often used in scenes about peer and social pressure.
- **The Protective Role:** This role portrays extreme emotional defenses, such as avoidance or denial, common to youth with developmental trauma. *The goal is for participants to become aware of the inner emotions that drive their behavior.*

Standard Theater Games

Theater games were initially designed to train actors. They were often used in rehearsal or the development of improvisation theater. Viola Spolin, an educator, acting teacher, and author of many books, including the well-known *Improvisation for the Theater,* created many theater games in 1963 that are still used today. Theater games generally teach team building, voice training, and communication skills. They are usually spontaneous and playful.[1]

The ENACT Application of Theater Games

ENACT has designed a framework for implementing theater games, delivered in phases, to build group trust and respond to the group's cognitive, emotional, and social needs. The games grow in intensity as the group can better handle them. The aim is to foster group cohesion and develop emotional safety while teaching skills based on the group's readiness level. ENACT theater games address behavior emotion regulation and teach coping skills.

For examples of theater games, see Chapter 7 and Appendices.

Monologue

In theater, a monologue is an uninterrupted speech in which a single character externalizes their innermost thoughts and feelings. It often "breaks the fourth wall" of the room we peer into when watching a scene, thus directly connecting with an audience. "To be or not to be" is a line from a famous dramatic monologue in Shakespeare's *Hamlet*. The monologue, which the actor delivers directly to the audience, depicts his deep internal struggles.

The ENACT Application of Monologue

A primary goal of the ENACT "inner monologue" is to externalize the core feelings hidden behind a character's defensive behavior.

For example, when communicating with another character in an ENACT scene, an actor expresses aggressive behavior, building to a conflict. A facilitator stops the scene, and, using the tool of inner monologue, the character faces the audience directly and reveals the thoughts and feelings hidden behind the behavior.

A typical inner monologue in an ENACT scene between an adolescent and their parent:

She doesn't understand me at all. Nobody understands me. I feel so alone. Sometimes, I feel like leaving, quitting school, and getting a job. I'm failing school anyway, so why bother? She gets me so angry; I'm not a child. I wish she understood me!

Core Therapeutic Concepts

The ENACT method is based on two core therapeutic concepts: **attachment** and **attunement**, and the two are closely connected. The quality of early attachment, whether it is positive or negative, affects the social, emotional, and mental health of a developing child. It can also affect their relationships throughout their life.

Attachment

Attachment refers to the early bond that develops in an emotionally healthy relationship between a child and a caregiver, offering them a secure base to grow. Children learn to regulate their emotions through interactions with their primary caregiver, which, with proper nurturing, allows them to feel safe and secure. When parents are reliable and offer comfort, children develop a secure sense of self.

An absent parent, neglect, or a lack of empathy from a parent to a child can cause **attachment rupture**. Without the safety needed to develop a healthy sense of self, children struggle to regulate their moods and emotions. Problems in self-regulation point to possible early attachment problems.

The good news is that caring adults offering positive relational experiences can provide corrective attachment experiences. ENACT offers these corrective experiences through a method built on a safe, reliable, emotional environment called a "creative container," explained in detail in Chapter 7. Signs of attachment rupture can often be seen in children and adolescents with behavior challenges stemming from problematic self-regulation. ENACT exercises are designed to help regulate emotions.

Attunement

Attunement is "a kinesthetic and emotional sensing of others, knowing their rhythm, affect and experience by metaphorically being in their skin, and going beyond empathy to create a two-person experience of unbroken feeling connectedness by providing a reciprocal affect and/or resonating response."[2] In other words, attunement means "tuning into" another person and responding to them without judgment.

Attunement is essential for working with youth with developmental trauma. For these teens, it is likely that their primary caregivers have never met their fundamental physical and emotional needs. As a result, they may have developed feelings of isolation that resulted in their emotional and behavioral challenges. They may never have had the benefit of a loving adult teaching them to regulate their emotions. These youth did not have the foundation to build trusting relationships with others.

Creative arts therapists use various innovative approaches to attunement, applying art, music, and dance approaches to build relationships with their clients and help them safely and indirectly connect with their emotions. They use their artistic tools to communicate and develop meaningful relationships that witness and affirm their client's process. The relationship can be a healing and a corrective experience for those who did not have their early attachment needs met.

Attunement is a child's primary communication with their caregiver. It is the key to forming and maintaining healthy relationships at the heart of positive attachment. When we genuinely attune with someone else, they feel seen and heard, which I believe can be translated into a representation of love. It is like a dance between two individuals, connecting move by move.

Being attuned to another provides a sense of being understood and cared about. A primary example of attunement might be an infant burbling their first sounds and a mother cooing the sounds back to them. The mother reflects her baby's feelings and expressions in a loving bond.[3]

Caregivers often don't realize that they "are out of tune." Concerned parents may worry about this, but missing the attunement boat occasionally is not as problematic as when an infant is chronically mis-attuned by their caregiver. Chronic negative attunement from a parent to a child can result in the child becoming disconnected from themselves, not reading or responding to their own needs. It is heartbreaking that when children are neglected, ignored, or abused, when attunement is not in the equation for them, they start out with less of a chance to regulate their emotions or form healthy relationships.

Empathetic Attunement

Empathetic attunement is key to the ENACT Method. It allows an actor/facilitator to take in the feelings and perceptions of the participants so they can reflect them back in a nonjudgemental way. It is a critical tool used by actors to create unspoken communication that can lead to a sense of bonding. The aim is to reflect behavior, needs, and experiences of the participants through characters they play in a scene. When individuals feel seen, heard and understood, it builds trust, and even the most resistant teens have proven to respond.

Embodied Attunement

ENACT uses **embodied attunement** in an intentional way to connect nonverbally with our participants. We use it to inform the creation and portrayal of the roles played in our scene work. The way it works: The actor "tunes into" one or more individuals in the room, feeling their way into their inner state, taking in their rhythm, tone, and intensity of the emotion. This internal "knowing" is then incorporated into the character they portray in the scene and reflected to the participants.

Like a tuning fork, embodied attunement is a form of interpersonal resonance. It is a very powerful means of connection that can spark self-reflection. **Note:** If, despite good intentions, the embodied attunement is off the mark, participants can feel mis-attuned, which can lead to resistance.

Mirroring

The ENACT role-play method is based on the concept of embodied attunement that uses **mirroring** to purposefully reflect the behaviors of others to encourage self-reflection. Mirroring describes the behavior when a person takes on another's gestures and emotions. It helps build a bridge between one person and another, bringing them into emotional unity. As Bessell van der Kolk explains, "Imitation is our most fundamental social skill. It ensures that we automatically pick up and reflect the behavior of our parents, teachers, and peers."[4]

Mirroring can demonstrate to another person that they are understood. It represents a form of validation that helps them feel their thoughts and feelings are accepted and worthwhile. Adolescents with trauma resulting from abuse and neglect rarely or never had their thoughts and feelings mirrored lovingly by their primary caregivers. This caused negative attachment. As a result, they developed feelings of being unworthy and unlovable. Since children cannot blame their caregivers for neglecting or mistreating them, they blame themselves instead, developing negative self-perceptions. "I must be bad if my parents don't love me." Through attunement, positive mirroring allows children and youth to see the good parts of themselves, an essential step in developing a more positive self-image.

Mirror Neurons

Mirroring is an automatic process, and it is the basis of empathy. The neurons involved in mirroring, known as mirror neurons, create internal maps of the internal states of others. As Dr. Daniel Siegel puts it, "Based on what we see in the world around us, mirror neurons may not only help us to imitate others' behaviors, but actually resonate with their feelings."[5]

The scientific discovery of mirror neurons in 1996 was groundbreaking. It showed how neurons found in the frontal and prefrontal lobes of the cortex allow the brain to imagine what another person is feeling or thinking. It is remarkable that our mirror neurons fire when we see others in action. It is as if we are doing the same thing. I believe that in the ENACT role-play, our process of embodied attunement is stimulating the mirror neurons in our observers.

Many creative arts therapists use experiential exercises to tap the mirror neurons of their clients to create connections as a first step toward healing. Arts educators and artists, although they may not be aware of mirroring as a concept, nonetheless use it through art forms such as drumming, chanting, movement, and improvisation, forming a verbal and nonverbal exchange with one another. These techniques have proven highly benefi-cial in helping teens with developmental trauma unearth their challenging feelings and accept vulnerable parts of themselves that have been pushed away. Meeting their protective layers through the creative act of mirroring allows them to feel safe enough to reflect on them.

Role-defense Mirroring

Adolescents who have suffered from neglect and abuse have developed layers and layers of protection, both physical and psychological. They become easily triggered if their protection is at risk of being compro-mised. They create defensive behavior for self-protection and survival. The result, unfortunately, may leave them disconnected from the self and unaware of their authentic thoughts and feelings. They may create a false self, wearing defenses like a coat of armor adorned with rigid pos-tures and defended attitudes.

Role-defense mirroring is an ENACT technique to join an individual by mirroring their behavior back to them. Actors portray a protected role within the safe context of a theatrical scene. They artfully play likable characters (so participants do not feel judged) with extreme behaviors embodying exaggerated posture, attitude, and language. Through observation, participants safely connect to the character without feeling exposed. Feeling seen and not judged develops trust. Hence, they become aware of their internal thoughts and feelings.

These core therapeutic concepts of attachment, attunement, and mir-roring are all essential tools for working with teens with developmental trauma. They can also be extremely powerful when working with other youth who feel alienated and isolated.

I offer below one of my favorite case histories, "The Moon Man," which was introduced at the start of this chapter.[6] While the popula-tion differed from the teens we generally served—this group was young children with autism—this story beautifully demonstrates the power of embodied attunement.

Now that I had come up with the metaphor of the lonely Moon Man, my next job was to come up with an activity. I needed to see if the group could focus on one exercise, follow directions, and interact with me or with each other. But most importantly, I needed to come up with an en-vironment that would allow their own expression to emerge—a *creative container* where change could happen. We needed to reflect a truth I had sensed about these children—that they were lonely and isolated—so that we could make a connection with them and let them know we knew how they felt. And that was when it came to me.

We'd take a trip to the moon.

"We're going on a journey," I told them. "We're going to visit a man on the moon. A Moon Man who is very sad. He's sad because no one understands him, and he can't speak our language." Bingo! We had a premise for connection. When I told the children we were taking a rocket to get there, they actually allowed us to gather them into a ragged line, our "rocket ship."

Taking our cue from young Jason's crash helmet, we encouraged everyone to hold on to their space helmets as we landed on the moon. We mimed slo-o-o-owly stepping over moon rocks, going under bridges, holding our noses so we could swim in moon-pools. Surprisingly, some of the children were able to do this—and we helped the ones who couldn't. As we journeyed toward the Moon Man, I whispered some directions in the ear of Brian, my colleague, and he disappeared behind the teacher's desk.

"Listen!" I told the group. "Do you hear something?" From behind the desk came a low moaning sound, a sound filled with longing. A purple shape gradually emerged from behind the "moon rock"—Brian, hunched over like a gentle Quasimodo, completely wrapped in purple fabric. Fascinated, every single child stood still to watch.

"The Moon Man is very shy," I told the children. "We have to move very slowly so we don't scare him."

So, slowly and carefully, I led the group toward the Moon Man, inviting each child to interact with him. The first little girl, Shawna, wanted to touch him. When she stood in front of the Moon Man, she gave a low laugh—and Brian echoed it. "Let's all do a quiet laugh," I suggested. Now completely engaged, the children laughed. Brian laughed, too.

"He's happy," I told them. "He knows we like him." The kids sure seemed to understand what I meant.

When it was his turn to see the Moon Man, Michael, the kinetic airplane boy I had noticed zooming around when we first entered the room, gave a little jump. Brian jumped, too. "Let's help the Moon Man to feel less lonely," I told the group. "Loud sounds and movements can scare him, so let's be very careful. Let's all jump!" Every child jumped to help the Moon Man. Michael made an inarticulate "U-h-h-h" sound. Then the Moon Man made an intuitive leap: He made a low sound—"I-I-I-I-I." Michael echoed it back. Then the Moon Man said "L-o-o-o-v-e." Incredibly, Michael repeated the word. Finally, the Moon Man said, "Y-o-o-o-u"—and so did Michael. This child, who was supposedly non-verbal, had said, "I love you." When the group echoed it back, I was stunned.

Without any prompting, Derek, the little boy in the big sweatshirt and pants, decided he wanted to give the Moon Man a gift. Solemnly, he handed an imaginary package to Brian, who mimed unwrapping it and then jumped up and down for joy. Derek jumped and laughed with delight. We all jumped up and down. After that, several other children wanted to give gifts to the Moon Man.

My eyes pricked with tears—only minutes before, these children, who had been in isolated worlds of their own, stood together, united in their intention to communicate love to another lonely being.

Afterward, Sally, the teacher, said, "I can't believe it. This is the first time I've ever heard any of these kids say a word. I didn't know they could even *make* words. And they've never shown such deep empathy for another person. I've never seen anything like it." We all agreed. For a few beautiful minutes, the children had come off of their lonely planets. All of our future work with youth of many ages and abilities would be a direct outgrowth of this important day.

Author's Notes

One question we are asked repeatedly—by parents, teachers, hospital workers, and others—is, "How can I reach a kid who won't talk to me? They turn off as soon as I open my mouth." Nonverbal children with autism can be seen as a kind of exaggerated version of the same withdrawal and alienation we often find in the typically abled youth population. However, because they are universal, the core principles and techniques that helped us reach this class of eight- and nine-year-olds will work just as effectively with older and/or less challenged youth.

- Attunement: We align with every individual we work with, feeling with mind, body, and soul, essence to essence. In this case, I was attuned to the feeling that I sensed in the youth: that they felt isolated and alone. That sparked my idea of taking them to the moon to meet another lonely being.
- Amazing things can happen when we find a way to express what someone feels—often, things they aren't even consciously aware of. Hearts can open, and healing can take place.

The great artist Michaelangelo once said that inside each stone, there was a beautiful figure waiting to be revealed, and his job was to use the right tools to free the truth that lay inside. All my years of working with young people have proved this to be true: Inside nearly every individual, no matter how troubled, is a human full of feelings, waiting to be released. The tools we need are connection, trust, empathy, and creativity.

Notes

1　Spolin, *Improvisation for the Theater.*
2　Erskine, *Int J Psychol.* 1998;3(3):235–244.
3　van der Kolk, *The Body Keeps the Score.* Quoting Beatrice Beebe, 120.
4　van der Kolk, *The Body Keeps the Score,* 114.
5　Siegel and Bryson, *The Whole-Brain Child,* 124.
6　Feldman, *Current Approaches in Drama Therapy.*

A Guide to the ENACT Drama Therapy Method

Chapter 6

Preparation

The five chapters in this section provide guidelines for implementing the ENACT Method in your work with teens. You can use this guidance to enhance and improve whatever methods you already employ, using principles you can apply to your work. You will also find theater games and other exercises here that will be beneficial. Training is recommended if you want to add the full version of ENACT to the services provided by your school, youth center, or hospital.

What ENACT Is

Using a unique combination of theater and drama therapy techniques, the ENACT Method aims to increase self-awareness as a first step to personal growth and change.

Through these techniques, including role-play and participatory theater games, practitioners of the ENACT Method can offer students alternative ways of perceiving themselves, behaving, and learning new life skills. The ENACT Method addresses relevant social issues that reflect the needs and concerns of students within a particular group, such as peer pressure, violence, and interpersonal conflicts. And because learning and change come from within, many of our activities are designed to tap inner awareness as a basis for creating personal and social change.

ENACT Principles

Before starting the process of setting up and implementing an ENACT workshop, it's important to understand its core principles. The following six principles form the methodology of ENACT.

DOI: 10.4324/9781003415022-9

1. See beyond the roles that teens present.

People are more than their obstacles, and it's important to see beyond those challenges. Each of us has an authentic self, a self that can be actualized. Within each of us is a creative essence that can be tapped into as a force for transformation.

2. Release judgment of self and others (develop compassion).

It is very easy to tell ourselves to release self-judgment, but we often spend time judging and criticizing ourselves. And what about the teens we work with? Do we judge them as well? These negative judgments do not serve our work; we can become more compassionate with others only if we start with ourselves. Physical, emotional, and academic obstacles can be dissolved if we look at what seems possible, as a foundation for learning.

3. Build relationships and create alliances.

Effective leadership and facilitation are essential in creating an opening for learning, growth, and change. For effective leadership to happen, a leader must build a strong working relationship with youth through attunement. A relationship based on truth, empathy, collaboration, and the pursuit of common goals creates an alliance between leaders and young people. Once an alliance is formed and a group feels attuned to, teens will be more willing to participate and take risks, enhancing the opportunities for self-awareness and positive change.

4. Transform via empowerment and validation.

Validation and empowerment are keys to change. When people feel good about themselves and know they are being acknowledged and heard (attuned to), they are more open to change. When they feel ashamed, they are more likely to retreat. A respectful relationship will be developed by an adult who makes it a habit to find the good in every student and reflect it back to them. When you do this, it is as though you are saying, "I see you as a human being with assets despite your obstacles, and we are here to work through the obstacles together."

For example, by telling Liam, who is acting up, that you understand how he may feel—and this does not mean you are allowing the behavior—you are allowing him to feel acknowledged *despite* his negative behavior. He will ultimately be more willing to redirect his actions than if you simply told him to stop and sit down. Charisse, on the other hand, may be terribly shy and withdrawn. She may not readily participate but will eventually come around and work with you if you respect her readiness level and validate her feelings.

5. Work developmentally (meet them where they're at).

Regularly assessing the group and individual needs can help you meet teens at their readiness level. It also assures them a sense of safety. Try to create or tailor exercises that match their age or functioning level. Age range and behavior are good initial factors to consider when creating exercises. For example, many teenagers hate to feel silly, especially in front of their peers, so choose games or tailor them to meet their developmental level. Adding just the right amount of challenge shows that you trust their ability. Adding too much challenge may set students up for failure. Student responses let you know, moment to moment, if the exercises are too simplistic or too challenging.

6. Teach accountability through limited choice and consequences.

Accountability is key to the ENACT work. To teach accountability, we introduce a limited choice, offering up three options in the classroom. For example, if a student does not seem interested and interrupts the workshop, they can participate without interrupting or sit out. They have a choice. Having limited choices allows teens to feel a sense of freedom and empowerment while learning to be accountable for their actions. It empowers them to become an integral part of creating a solution. It instills a sense of responsibility as students learn the consequences of their choices. We have found that using choice and natural consequences to teach accountability is the most effective way of improving behavior.

The magic of the ENACT Method lies in its preplanned design, delivered by highly engaging facilitators and actors who perform scenes relevant to the group's lives. So before you engage with students directly, take the following steps to prepare.

Gather the Necessary Information

An initial assessment is essential to designing an effective workshop, customized and delivered by two skilled facilitators.

To conduct an initial assessment, an ENACT facilitator meets with the person in charge of the youth program. This person could be a school principal, teacher, or social worker, but it must be someone who knows the kids. The assessment informs the facilitator about the environment where participants live, individual needs, and behavior. It can include specific details of group members' likes and dislikes, down to subtleties such as the food in the cafeteria or a significant event that happened in recent weeks or even that day. You can create your own questions, depending on the participants you're working with.

Needs Assessment Questionnaire: Suggested Subjects and Questions

- **The environment.** *This information allows the scene to be designed within a context the young people can relate to.*

  – What are the living situations/contexts of the teens in the group? Do some teens live in one-parent homes, public housing, or foster care?
  – Please describe the neighborhoods where the teens live, including factors such as levels of crime or the potential that they might witness acts of violence, including police violence.

- **The statistics.** *Helps in designing the activities and selecting the actors.*

  – What is the age, gender, pronouns, and culture of the group?

- **The behavior.** *Helps shape the goals of the theater games, i.e., to help regulate behavior. Initial information about the behavior also allows the actors to approximate an imitation of their behavior, which will become more accurate as they observe and get to know the participants.*

  – What brings you to seek the ENACT work?
  – What are the youth's primary challenging behaviors? Rebellious? Apathetic? Antagonistic? Something else? How is the group dynamic?
  – Please describe the expression of the behavior.
  – Have you noticed any specific triggers for these behaviors? What are they?

- **Likes and dislikes.** *Allows facilitators to demonstrate that they under-stand the group. Planting specific information in the scenario for them to recognize, such as an event that happened that day or what they had for lunch, helps them feel seen and heard, which goes a long way in building group trust.*

  – What does the group like or dislike about the environment?
  – Are there any current events to be aware of?

Based on the information gathered, theater games and relevant scenes will be designed to foster self-awareness, teach coping skills, and encourage social-emotional learning. This information enables facilitators to create lessons that foster engagement, build group trust, and, most of all, lead the group members to form alliances that encourage personal insights.

Sometimes, facilitators may be asked to address specific issues disrupting the group, such as bullying or teasing. There may be an issue of collective trauma that is affecting the entire school, being felt but not expressed by a group, affecting their ability to communicate. After 9/11, for example, New York City students were so traumatized they could not speak about it, and the indirect method of creative drama helped them to express their feelings.

The goal of every session is to have an engaged, cohesive group that takes part in an interactive learning process designed to help teens gain insight into behaviors and underlying emotions. This leads to a process of change.

While many of the teens ENACT worked with would greatly benefit from therapy, it was my experience that most of them would refuse help in this format if it were offered to them directly. ENACT's process occurs through theater and acting, which engages teens in a therapeutic process often without them knowing it. Still, when ENACT encountered a new group, members often resisted participating in even this type of therapeutic process, but they eventually joined in.

The first step is to address the resistance by helping teens feel seen, heard, and respected. This is accomplished by creating lessons they resonate with, to hook them into the process, often weaving specific details of their lives into the lesson plan's central activity (the facilitator's scene work). Once the group feels seen and understood, they are drawn into participating in a deepening process. Engagement and participation are likely.

Adjust the Assessment as Needed

While information is gathered at the start of the ENACT process, assessment is built into every ENACT activity. Instructors can adjust activities to meet the group's ever-changing dynamics. Group leaders observe and respond to the group's social interactions, affect level, and individual responses. Theater games are adjusted to meet the group's tolerance levels. The group leader observes resistance levels rising or falling based on responses to an activity and adjusts accordingly. ENACT activities have the benefit of simultaneously assessing a group and teaching skills.

For example, when facilitators notice that a group is becoming increasingly resistant to the activities, asking what is going on is a form of in-the-moment assessment. Common adolescent statements such as "this is boring" or "this is stupid," while initially discouraging, provide invaluable feedback that suggests an activity is too easy or difficult for them. An increase or decrease in the game's level of challenge or changing the activity to meet the group's needs could be effective responses.

Cast the Players

Every ENACT session is co-led by two facilitators. There are several reasons why it's important to have two people if this is at all possible. The most obvious is that they improvise with each other in the scene work. Another important reason is that they can support each other to manage the class. This is particularly important if the the majority of the students become easily dysregulated. While one teaches the lesson, the other concentrates on keeping the class focused. This is important because the groups we worked with could easily become triggered and interfere with the process.

One facilitator is designated as the group leader, and the other is a group supporter. The group leader is often a mental health practitioner or skilled educator; the supporter is an actor adept at improvisation. The group leader is responsible for creating a safe experience for youth supported by their peers. The supporter is responsible for working with individuals in the group if they become distracted, dysregulated, show distress, or divert attention from the group's cohesiveness during activities. If only one practitioner is available, it is helpful to invite another adult, such as the classroom teacher or even a willing student, to join you.

One or both facilitators should reflect the group's ethnicity and culture. If, for example, the group consists of primarily Latinx boys with acting-out behavior, we would try to select a Latinx actor who speaks Spanish and can portray an aggressive role. Reflecting on a group's culture and behavior in a role-play helps youth feel attuned and can immediately reach even the most resistant youth. Factors like humor, compassion, and of course, expertise are also important when selecting actors and facilitators because their skills help to build trust, safety, and connection.

The Leader

The leader exhibits confidence and leads with compassion. They are responsible for setting the tone and creating the workshop environment. The first impression is very important, and that is why the first session, in particular, must be carefully conducted. The leader lays the foundation, creates the atmosphere, and explains the guidelines. They are creating the structure of the entire workshop, with a clear beginning, middle, and end. It is essential for the leader to know their objective for each exercise and to stay aware of what they are trying to achieve.

As the leader guides the lesson, they must be clear that they are in charge and "holding the reins," especially in the beginning. As the group develops trust, they can loosen the reins, little by little. Although a lesson plan may move in unexpected directions based on the group's responses and needs, the leader will need to bring the workshop back to a clear closure that reinforces the theme. A good leader is like an orchestra conductor, guiding the pace and rhythm of the group as a whole while allowing for solo expression. An effective leader manages and monitors the flow, tone and affect levels of the group.

A good leader must...

Read the room.

As a leader, when I meet a group for the first time, I open myself up to take the room's temperature. First, I observe the entire group dynamic, and then I scan the individuals in the group to get a sense of who may be highly acting out, resistant, etc. This immediate impression helps me deliver my lesson based on who is in the group. The environment as a whole must be considered when implementing a lesson. The activities may only be successful when the person is aware of the moment-to-moment feeling in the room. Therefore, the leader must read the room from the moment they walk in.

This takes time and experience. As you become more relaxed, this will happen naturally. Practice trusting your inner self as you do activities, and soon you will respond on a moment-to-moment basis. It is the key to becoming a strong and intuitive leader. You will also find that as you do so, you will enjoy the process even more.

Create group cohesion.

A primary goal for a group leader is to create group cohesion. Working well together as a group encourages a feeling of belonging and connection, especially for those who tend to isolate. It supports risk-taking, joint decision-making, and accomplishing group tasks.

Allow room for your intuition.

How can we respond with a creative idea or reaction just when it is needed? How do we sense who we should focus on at the right moment? Your intuition can play a big role during the sessions—if you allow it. When you are focused on your intention, an exercise or idea may come to you in the moment. Trust that. It is fine to move in unexpected directions, veering away from the lesson plan, if you keep the lesson's goal in mind and ultimately bring it back into focus. There are times when, based on group response and discussion, you decide the goal for the workshop is changing. This is okay as long as the new goal has clear outcomes attached to it and the group is clear about where they are going and what they are learning. Working intuitively develops over time, through experience, trust, and competence. In fact, there are times when the true goal will present itself as it emerges from the group, and your job is simply to reshape the lesson. Even so, it is recommended that you always design an initial lesson plan. If you tend to work intuitively, it is especially important to establish a strong working relationship with your partner so that they can support you in each moment.

Establish predictability.

Being predictable creates safety and structure. Participants should become familiar with the ENACT workshop ritual of a "beginning," usually theater games; "middle," usually role-play; and "end, "which offers feel-good closures. In ongoing workshops, repeating games, such as group rhythm and movement, allows for the predictability needed by participants.

Regulate the energy flow.

The leader must regulate the flow of energy in the room as though it had a knob like a radio. If the energy level is too high and the class gets out of hand, the leader must bring the energy level down. If, on the other hand, the energy level is too low and the students are apathetic, the leader must turn the knob up a few notches and raise the group's energy.

Acknowledge the transitions.

Although there may be stopping and starting during a session, the leader can keep things flowing by including transitions between the exercises. Transitions are essential to a good session. With appropriate transitions, exercises can feel connected to the group response.

So, how do we make these transitions? Once an exercise is over, what do you do? Some exercises flow gently from one to the next, while others need a few moments of silence to center the group's energy. Consider inviting students to take a few breaths or to shake out excess energy before beginning a new activity. Listening to responses and feeling group energy will help you know how to segue into the next exercise.

Understand enactment, not re-enactment.

Be mindful that during certain exercises, especially in role-plays, teens who have experienced trauma may want to reenact an incident. It's their way of making sense of a situation and trying to resolve the trauma. However, *re-enacting a trauma is not what will heal the trauma.* For example, in a workshop in a juvenile justice center, a group of teens wanted to act out an incident of a drive-by shooting they witnessed in their neighborhood. They all wanted to re-enact the incident and play the part of the shooter. After a few replays, we saw that the group was becoming highly activated, hyper-aroused, in a way that was not productive. To maintain control and safety, we redirected them to another activity. When teens want to play out the original trauma repetitively in a role-play, you can offer them other safer opportunities to express their feelings.

Support accomplishment every step of the way.

For individuals who have experienced trauma, experiencing a sense of mastery is important for their healing. This is because experiencing trauma can make them feel helpless. Allowing them to master an activity, like a theater game, is invaluable to them. ENACT exercises are designed to be strength-based, and celebrating achievements of individuals and the group as a whole can be achieved by adding a round of applause after each exercise and, when appropriate, having an awards ceremony at the end of a program.

The leader should keep these questions in mind:

- Have I set the tone?
- Am I attuning with the group?
- Am I sticking to the goal or theme of the day? Why or why not?
- Is there group cohesion?
- Am I responding to the group energy through proper transitions?
- Am I regulating the energy level?
- Am I communicating with my partner?

Acknowledge separation and loss.

It is worth reiterating that adolescence is a time of intense change. During this phase, it is essential to remember that a connection with caring adults is critical to them. If an adolescent experiences a broken bond in a meaningful relationship with an adult, which could be you, it can create an onset of earlier traumatic memories from early attachment wounds.

Early on in my drama therapy work with youth groups, I experienced a teen's reaction to loss. It happened at the end of my drama therapy program, working with middle school students in Brooklyn. It was a tough group. After several weeks of wrestling with their resistance and unruly behavior, we finally built cohesion and trust. We accomplished a lot of creative therapeutic work.

In the last session, after my closure activity, I said goodbye to the group, knowing we would not see each other again. As I began to exit, a student ran up to me, started crying uncontrollably, saying, "Don't leave," and held on to me so tightly that I couldn't get out of her grip. The teacher had to pull her away. As I walked out the door, I looked back and saw the expression on the young teen's face; she looked so sad and felt terrible. The idea that I could have hurt her in my attempts to help felt awful.

When I left the room, I realized that even though the adolescents seemed so tough and infallible, what I was witnessing were defenses that were protecting their vulnerability. I also realized that leaving too abruptly without addressing the feelings of separation and loss could trigger old memories of loss and breaches in relationships. Avoiding the elephant in the room was a mistake. Many of these adolescents suffered from attachment wounds, and I should have been more aware that the group needed time to process feelings before I left.

Attachment wounds are common with youth who have experienced trauma, so keep in mind that your relationship with them matters more than you think. Separation is a sensitive issue for many youth with trauma histories despite their tough exterior, so connection and separation must be handled with great care.

ENACT has developed a series of closure activities and affirmations to honor and address feelings of loss. Some of our scenarios broached the topic of loss by doing distanced scenes relating to friends moving or going away to college. This opened up discussions around much deeper issues. Prepare for a final meeting or session prepared with various tools.

Techniques for Managing Trauma Caused by Separation and Loss

- Understand the gravity of loss for youth with attachment wounds.
- Let individuals know up front when your sessions will be over.
- Communicate your feelings about leaving.
- Allow discussions on separation and loss.
- Discuss how to hold on to good feelings and memories.
- Take a photograph of the group and leave it with them to commemorate their time together.

The Supporter

The supporter's role is just as important as that of the leader. The supporter is focused on the individual needs of each student. They monitor those needing extra help, redirection, or assurance and offer it in a supportive way. For example, suppose the supporter notices an individual undermining the group with negative behavior. They might ask the individual to step out of the circle and help them one-on-one with emotional regulation until they feel ready to join the group again. In this way, the supporter is helping the leader by removing a significant distraction while also helping the student to regroup.

The supporter must be aware of everything that the leader must do to maintain group cohesion. This is especially important because sometimes the supporter is called upon to co-lead an activity.

Supporters should be aware of the following responsibilities:

Be encouraging.

Gently go around the circle to see if the participants follow the leader's directions. Keep bringing focus to the leader. Do not draw attention to yourself. Reinforce what the leader is doing and check on individual needs. If someone is stuck, help them out; if someone is making noise, ask them to be quiet, etc. The supporter maintains the guidelines set up by the leader. The management of the classroom often depends on a strong supporter.

Intervene when necessary.

If a student is distracting the group and making it difficult for the lesson to continue, you should intervene. Talk to that student or take them aside (or, if necessary, out of the room) and speak with them privately. Once that student is made aware of their behavior, help them regulate their emotions with mindful breathing and counting. You can also give them choices that are in service to them and to the rest of the group, such as the option to remove themselves from the activity. Stand next to the disruptive or withdrawn student and encourage positive participation.

Be prepared to respond immediately to an activity or intervention indicated by the leader.

> **The supporter should keep these questions in mind:**
>
> • Am I supporting my partner on an "as-needed" basis?
> • Am I helping to maintain the structure and boundaries of the session?
> • Am I helping to address individual needs in support of the group?

Design the Lessons

The group leader is the lesson plan's architect and implementer, although both instructors collaborate on planning the activities. Based on the assessment and after initial observation, the group leader carries out a customized plan for each session with every group. They select or create theater games and design scenes based on the group's needs to reach specific goals for each session.

For a lesson plan to be effective, it must be designed with specific objectives. However, the ENACT Method is an art more than a science. Any good plan may get tossed out once the group session begins because the session must be responsive to the group's moment-to-moment needs. For example, the plan for that session may have been the goal of students having the group learn specific social and emotional skills, such as relationship skills; however, if the behavior of the group is particularly reactive that day, activities may need to change to work on self-regulation skills.

Some stock ENACT scenes have proven particularly effective as attention grabbers for the youth. For example, a scene about The Class Clown who becomes triggered when the teacher calls him out on his behavior is usually successful. The role of The Class Clown demonstrates the student's silly behavior as a defense against his inner feelings of sadness and his reactive aggressive behavior when triggered by the teacher. Another relatable scene was a parent telling their child that they cannot go to a party, and the teen becomes furious. Most of the students we worked with could relate to these defenses, the triggers, or both. The character of the teen would be likable, so the students would not feel judged.

When we present an initial scene like this, we have two goals. The first is to engage the students so they will be willing to participate in the deeper work. The second is to use the scene as a form of assessment, listening deeply to how individuals respond to the processing activity following the scene. We tune in to what students say and don't say and how they react. This not only gives us information about the group as a whole, but about individuals we may need to focus on.

How the Lessons Are Structured

The ENACT process has three phases: the warm-up, the main activity, and the closure. Each complements the other two. The following three chapters will describe these phases in more detail. For now, here is an overview.

Phase 1: The Warm-Up

The warm-up generally consists of theater games, usually running for approximately 15 minutes. It uses engaging, playful theater games to encourage creativity and spontaneity through rhythm, sound, and movement. It is often linked to the goals of the main activity and prepares the group for the next phase, the upcoming scene work.

Phase 2: The Main Activity

The main activity, which is usually the most extended phase of the session, consists of the role-play/inquiry process. Depending on the allocated session time, it can last 30–40 minutes.

The main activity has two parts.

- Part one demonstrates *a real life scenario reflective of common youth experiences and performed by the actors* that mirrors the behaviors and feelings of the participants. As participants resonate with the scenario, they feel safe to engage in a deepening process of self-reflection through an inquiry process aimed at helping them gain personal insights into unspoken parts of themselves.
- Part two *invites participants to replay the scene using various alternatives.* It is used for skill building and is the most extended phase of the session. It consists of scene work and an inquiry phase aimed at helping youth gain insight into the underlying emotions that cause their reactive behavior. Through the safe distance of theater, youth examine their thoughts, feelings, and behaviors. They are invited to replay the scene with their new-found skills.

Phase 3: The Closure

The closure is usually the same length as the warm-up or can be shorter, depending on the available time left for the session. The closure is a completion of the workshop using embodied activities to help youth integrate what they have learned and imprint it with their bodies and minds.

Note: A specific amount of time should be allocated for each phase, but stay flexible. The group may need more time in one phase or another, depending on the needs of that day. Time frames can be adjusted to ensure that the session ends on time. Routine is essential for youth, especially if they have experienced trauma. Consistency offers a sense of safety and can act as an anchor for them.

Tips for Designing the Session

It's important to think about the group when designing these phases. You collected information about the students in the initial gathering phase. Now you can use it. Also, take into consideration the following:

1. **Know the time allocation of the session** so you can plan phases accordingly.

2. **Know the space you will occupy** to set up the creative working space within it.

    You will often work within an institution such as a school or hospital where an adult is in charge. Plan to align with this person by involving them actively (inviting them to join the session) or passively (asking them to keep notes and give you feedback). Form a relationship with them as you do with your youth. Your relationship with this person will be important to the program's success.

3. **Plan for addressing behavior.** If you were told that the group members are very reactive and explosive, you should assume that they may have experienced developmental trauma, causing issues of trust. Assume that you will be met with resistance when working to engage them in the process. You should do something to engage them immediately to create interest and willingness. You can start with a solid, reflective (nonjudgmental) sample scene of an explosive student in a conflict with a teacher, a peer, or a parent. This is often the hook to invite them into the process. Give them an out by offering them an option to not participate or to "pass." Since these teens may become easily triggered, plan strength-based theater games, allowing for success and use of games for containment and regulation. The supporter should plan to be ready to work with disruptive youth outside the main area to support the containment of the group.

Social and Emotional Skills and Coping Skills You Will Teach

There are many skills that can be developed by those who engage in the ENACT Method, and this list can be useful in helping you design your sessions. This list evolved over many years of working with students of various ages and abilities.

Emotion-Regulation Skills

Students will:

- Learn coping skills such as control over impulses (i.e., able to control behavior, sit or stand silently for 10 seconds, slow down, relax, think before acting).
- Learn to differentiate between behavior and core needs.
- Learn self-regulation skills include breathing, counting to 10, self-talk, and walking away when all else fails.
- Learn the value of exercise, guided imagery, and relaxation methods.
- Practice grounding techniques like the *butterfly hug* and meditation.
- Practice self-advocating (ask for help when needed).

Social and Emotional Skills

Students can:

- Articulate and understand feelings.
- Name feelings.
- Express their feelings constructively.
- Recognize behaviors.
- Learn decision-making skills.
- Develop relationship skills.
- Develop conflict-resolution skills.
- Understand others' feelings and concerns and accept their perspective.

Next up: how to run the session itself.

Chapter 7

Phase I: The Warm-Up (Theater Games)

ENACT worked in a high school in Jamaica, Queens, in the early nineties. We were placed in a special education classroom for a double period once a week for an entire year. The students in this classroom were labeled "acting out," meaning they displayed reactive behavior and had issues with attendance. Then there was Lamont, a tall, large young man with a childlike face and awkward gait who always carried a lollipop and a comb in his back pocket. He was very likable, and also very challenging.

The first day was relatively easy. We played theater games but noticed immediately that the group had difficulty focusing. They would get distracted by noises outside the classroom and loud PA (public address) announcements. They would also get distracted by their teacher or each other. Some of the teens seemed to be off in their own worlds, and I often had to redirect them. I didn't understand it then, but I now know that they exhibited signs of hypervigilance.

Lamont, on the other hand, would suck on his lollipop or comb his hair and continually interrupt the process. He was highly reactive to the teacher, but the other students didn't seem to mind and accepted his outbursts. They enjoyed the exercises, but we were planning to work there for a year, so we needed to find a way for them to stay involved and attend class.

We decided to work toward a culminating performance, and at our next session, I suggested the idea to them. They were excited about the prospect of being on stage, so we had their buy-in, which would be a carrot for their mandated attendance; we told them that regular attendance was one of the main criteria for participating in the final performance. But that day, I noticed someone missing. It was Lamont.

DOI: 10.4324/9781003415022-10

You may be working with groups anywhere from days to weeks to months or a full year. In the case history that begins above, we were working with the students for several months. (You will read the rest of Lamont's story later in this chapter.) In cases like this, it's important to plan each session as well as to plan a project to keep teens engaged for a longer-term process. At ENACT, we often created culminating performances.

Once you have completed your prep work, it's time to meet the teens and interact. You are ready for the first part of the ENACT session in which you will "warm up" the participants by engaging them in theater games. The warm-up usually runs for about 15 minutes and will prepare the participants for the transformative process of scene work in the main activity.

First Impressions

The Greeting

As we all know, first impressions count. Upon entering the room for the first time, introduce yourself (if the participants don't already know you) and consider greeting everyone separately. Smile or shake their hand, saying a positive word or two. From my experience, I have learned that an individual greeting is invaluable. It provides your first opportunity to earn trust. Some youth you work with will have trauma histories. Remember that trauma often renders individuals wary, and developing trust may take some time. Inviting them into the play space by offering them a choice instead of coercing them is the first step in building a trusting relationship.

Introduce and Explain the Guidelines

Explain that this workshop has a policy created to help everyone feel safe. You might introduce it like this: "We will do some acting in this workshop. Actors explore various emotions, and we will, too. To feel safe, we need the help of the group. We will all be taking creative risks that need support. Let's discuss what it means to support someone." In your discussion, include that all ENACT exercises are followed with a round of applause.

Respect Resistance

Use the Pass Directive

Participants can opt out or declare "pass" on any activity that makes them feel uncomfortable. This concept represents respect for the autonomy of its participants, and it's a good idea to introduce this to participants when they first meet you. You might say, "If you are uncomfortable about doing an exercise, you can say 'pass,' which means you can opt out of the exercise as long as you support the group."

When a participant uses a pass, the choice is to be respected as conscious and responsible rather than resorting to defensive behavior. The use of "pass" avoids or diminishes resistance upfront. Of course, participants are regularly invited to participate in the process for the following activities.

Introduce Partial Gaze

For exercises in which you ask students to close their eyes, always offer the alternative of students keeping their eyes open or in an partial gaze. Students who have experienced trauma often prefer to keep their eyes open or in a half gaze.

Create the Physical Space

Set up the space to be as comfortable as possible. If you can, rearrange the room so students are removed from their usual atmosphere. Push back the chairs or desks and have them stand, forming a circle where everyone works equally. If the chairs cannot be moved, simply create the space by pulling down an imaginary curtain to welcome students to the workshop space.

Wherever you are—and it may be in a gym, a cafeteria, an auditorium, or even a large bathroom (this actually happened to me once)—it is essential to create a contained space. If you don't, especially in the larger spaces, students may easily wander and this can compromise the safety of the space.

Most important: Try to arrange the room based on the group dynamic. If there is a lot of chaos in the room, you may need to start with students staying in their seats. We usually work in a circle. It's also recommended that you place a note on the door to let passersby know that a workshop is in progress.

A Safe Environment: The "Creative Container"

As we've already discussed, adolescents with chronic trauma get triggered easily. Trauma severs trust and takes away a sense of control, and often, youth feel helpless. It's our job to help them feel safe and protected.

ENACT interventions work with youth to lessen this sense of violation by providing safety, reliability, social support, empowerment, and peer connections. We provide what we call the **creative container**.

The creative container is like a social system, a microcosm designed to build social support through a community experience that has predictable boundaries. It is also a physical space established during ENACT sessions, where activities are usually conducted in a circle representing unity and where expressive activities like rhythm, movement, and sound act as healing rituals. The container can be set up almost anywhere—in classrooms, hospital standard rooms, and youth centers—creating physical and emotional boundaries.

Within the safe container, the group leader takes on the role of a theater director who, like any creative director, uses specific techniques to maintain the structure and flow and transitions from activity to activity. Youth are supported by peers who witness their courage to take risks. The space allows for the safe expression of thoughts, perceptions, and feelings.

The container is a therapeutic space that respects every individual's potential, offering opportunities for self-awareness and transformation.

An ENACT program evaluator team funded by the Ford Foundation characterized the creative container as "a space that values the human spirit and provides emotional boundaries that neither overwhelms emotions nor distances them, a key factor that impedes learning."[1]

Within this container, customized theater games and other dramatic activities are carried out to promote expression and spontaneity, often absent from the lives of youth with trauma whose internal lives may be confining and rigid. Activities usually progress from highly structured to less structured as the group develops trust, safety, and confidence. Sometimes contracts of agreement are designed, especially recommended for adolescents with behavior challenges.

More on Keeping Things Safe

ENACT developmental theater games are designed to meet individuals "where they are" emotionally, physically, and cognitively. They are strength-based and build self-confidence as they prepare participants for the next level of challenge.

Theater games are adjusted to help participants feel confident in taking creative risks. Facilitators start with a high level of structure and slowly loosen the reins, allowing for greater spontaneity once the group develops cohesion and confidence.

Youth are willing to participate in an activity when it is engaging and fun and the group feels safe and supportive enough for them to take risks. But when teens feel unsafe or uncomfortable, they will voice their dislike and may do so directly.

Teens' responses to games should be read as signals about their level of emotional safety and are expressed to protect them from feeling inadequate.
Participants are never to be blamed, even if their behavior is challenging.
They are your partners in a give-and-take process.

Developmental theater games are also designed to minimize feelings of shame, an essential goal when working with teens. Adolescents, as they individuate from their parents or caregivers, are highly tuned into their peer groups' impressions of them and often go to great lengths to impress them. Peer support is essential to the group because teens take risks by trying new activities and experimenting with roles. Teens must feel the leader has set up a protective, *shame-free zone* and is their ally. A facilitator achieves this by disallowing judgment and criticism from anyone in the group. Validation is always encouraged as a regular source of feedback, and group applause after activities demonstrates a sense of accomplishment.

Creating a Contract with the Participants

It is often helpful for the facilitator to create a written contract with the participants and signed by them, especially when dealing with adolescents with challenging behavior. *This is not something that is done at the first session.* A contract should only be created once the students are willing to participate in the workshop, whether the workshop takes place over a week, a month, or a year. A contract establishes agreements about how to keep the creative container safe. It encourages accountability.

Within this contract, consequences must be established to reinforce the goal of group safety and cohesion. It's important to note that the consequences are not punitive; they are about accountability. They encourage the best in people. The facilitators might introduce the notion of consequences democratically by saying something such as, "We all slip up once in a while, including me, so what should we do if this happens?"

After soliciting ideas for group agreements from the participants, I recommend you suggest a "three-strikes-and-you're-out" policy.

Say something like, "Instead of someone getting kicked out of the circle right away, what if we get three chances and then are asked to leave the activity until the next one begins and they are ready to try again? Does that sound fair?"

The "three-strikes" technique is effective because it works in stages. The idea is that after the contract is designed with the class and ritualized by signing it and hanging it in view of all, it should be enforced.

The leader does not need to be the enforcer. In fact, it is better if the students do it, but it must be done in a supportive way. I suggest to the students that there will be two verbal warnings when the contract is violated. On the third warning, they will be asked to leave the working area, although they are invited back to try again after an appropriate period. In this way, it becomes a challenge—not a punishment—for students to work on their behavior and become accountable.

When negotiating a contract, work democratically so students feel they are part of the process and not coerced into it. Solicit suggestions from students when setting up the contract. Contracts may vary from group to group depending on the class dynamic and lesson goals. By the way, the facilitators should also be held accountable for following the agreements in the contract.

Sample Contract

In this workshop, we agree to:
Be respectful.
Be supportive.
Have no invasive physical contact (pushing, hitting).
Use appropriate language.
Take chances.
Be on time.
Be at every session.
Try our best.
Have fun!

To illustrate how creating a contract made a big impact on a group, we return to the case history started at the beginning of this chapter, about Lamont, the big kid with the lollipop.[2]

The behavior of the group was clearly challenging. So, in addition to dangling the carrot of an eventual theatrical performance, we also created a group contract. "So, what would help you feel comfortable in this creative process?" I asked. As students called out their answers, "no hitting," "no lying," and "no teasing," I wrote them down on the blackboard. "How about we create a group contract that we all sign?" I suggested. They agreed, and we created a contract with a three-strikes-and-you-are-out policy. They all signed it, and I hung it up on the board.

We raised the stakes even more and told them the performance would occur at an Off-Broadway theater. Since many of them had never been to the theater, I described what it would be like and told them I would arrange a visit ahead of time. They were excited.

We started to create the show by coming up with topics they wanted to address, such as peer pressure and bullying. We began working on scenes for the first few days. But Lamont was still not showing up.

Then one day, Lamont strolled into the classroom late, armed with headphones and his usual lollipop. "What happened to you, Lamont? We missed you." Lamont looked at me with a childlike expression. He had missed the previous days when we had discussed our agreements.

As the program progressed, Lamont continued to push the limits of the class. He continued to show up late, interrupt, and crack jokes. He had a way of creating chaos. Each day was a struggle. He had difficulty relating to the other students; he broke every rule set by the group. We spent a great deal of time redirecting and channeling his creative energy into the work. Lamont was also an excellent actor. He had a natural gift. However, he needed to attend class regularly, not just when he felt like it. How could we get Lamont to contain his behavior and use his acting ability to strengthen our show?

The group was bonding, and the play was shaping up despite Lamont's rare attendance. However, one day, when we were all sitting in a circle, one of the students suggested we kick him out of the show. We all knew that Lamont liked the acting process and felt it would be unfair to discuss kicking him out without him there. In the middle of our discussion, Lamont showed up, wanting to know what we were talking about. The students discussed our contract with him and told him we wanted him in the show, but we could only continue if he followed the rules and showed up regularly. He listened, and his childlike face looked sad.

"What's going on, Lamont?" I asked. He said he was having a hard time at home and knew he was having difficulty controlling himself. Lamont pleaded with us to let him stay, and one of the students suggested we revisit the contract, adding being on time, not interrupting, and, most of all, having fun. They explained the three-strikes-and-you-are-out clause. We drafted a new contract and hung it on the wall. Lamont signed it. He agreed that after three warnings, he and anyone else who was being disruptive (even accidentally) had to sit out of the circle until they were ready to participate productively with the group. If they continued to disrupt, they would have to leave.

Lamont messed up a few times, and so did we all. But he reined in his behavior and even stepped out of the circle himself before he was asked to. He owned his behavior and even apologized to the group for disrupting. Lamont was becoming accountable for his behavior. He showed up every day and worked hard. We continued to acknowledge his efforts and successes. The group had a very positive effect on him; he felt supported and recognized for his strengths. Lamont positively impacted the group as they observed him become consciously aware of his behavior, trying to regulate and own its effect on the group. The show was shaping up and getting close to being performed. The group's excitement was rising, and so was their anxiety. Each day we did calming exercises, including breathing and guided visualizations.

The big night was here, and enthusiastic friends and family sat in the audience. Backstage, everyone was holding hands and saying a prayer. Afterwards, Lamont told the group that no one in his family was in the audience. We acknowledged his disappointment and sadness. I told Lamont that we were like a substitute family.

The lights went up, the students stepped on stage, and Lamont, who had become a lead in the show, shined. In the discussion following the performance, the students sat on the stage. An audience member said, "You were remarkable!" Another asked, "How did you work so well as a group?" Lamont responded, admitting, "At first, it wasn't easy, but we all really tried." We all laughed. Lamont came through with shining colors, empowered with new self-awareness, and bonded with a community of peers.

Author's Notes

- This group of students demonstrated several symptoms of trauma, from hypervigilance–expressed through their heightened awareness of stimuli–to signs of dissociation, as they seemed to go off in their own worlds.
- Lamont found ways to self-soothe using his lollipop and comb to calm himself.
- The group was a healing force for Lamont as they redirected his behavior and were there for him when his family was not.
- The group contract was very effective, and the students reinforced the consequences.

Theater Games

Bottom-Up Activities

ENACT warm-up activities are centered around theater games. These games are rooted in **embodiment techniques**. Embodiment involves the interaction of the body with thoughts and feelings. This is also referred to as a bottom-up approach. When individuals gain a greater awareness of their bodies and how they react to others, they can recognize the feelings stored inside.

Once students recognize those feelings, they are encouraged to express them, and a transformation process begins. Drama therapist and professor Renée Emunah explains, "When the beginning exercises allow group members to express actual feelings, defenses are minimized."[3] She goes on to say, "With this approach to drama therapy, clients have little to resist because they are allowed to act as themselves."

ENACT theater games purposefully integrate body-mind through movement, rhythm, sound, and embodied expression, facilitating growth and healing. They also teach emotion regulation, self-awareness, and self-efficacy.

The games can also be used to address emotion regulation:

- *Grounding exercises ease anxiety (hyperarousal).* Examples of grounding exercises are breathing and internal counting.
- *Stimulating exercises lift low mood (hypoarousal or depression),* incorporating dance and rhythm.
- *Improvisational exercises reduce the overactivity of the mind and encourage impulse control,* focusing on challenging activities.

Spontaneity, play, and creative expression allow teens to become fully present as they explore thoughts and feelings often repressed in those who have experienced trauma. The field of trauma recognizes that trauma lives in the body, and growing evidence points to the importance of body-based approaches ("bottom-up" experiences) for healing. A supportive environment allows for risk-taking while teens build interpersonal relationships and connections.

Basic Theater-Based Commands

Before the interactive portion of the session begins, the facilitator explains various commands that will be used from time to time. Acting as a theater director, the facilitator introduces commands like "freeze," "focus," and "center." They practice them with the participants to assure safety and maintain group cohesion.

The leader delivers these commands as supportive and playful challenges, and participants should enjoy responding. The leader can deliver the commands whenever the group loses focus, gets out of control, or becomes too activated, compromising the group's integrity.

Freeze Command

"Freeze" is a command introduced to stop the action when needed during a group activity to direct participants to freeze in position when they hear it called out. This directive is used when the group becomes too activated, loses focus, gets out of control, and needs to return to a neutral stance. This directive is especially beneficial to children and youth with impulse control issues because it helps them self-regulate. The leader calls "freeze" and "unfreeze" at any time in the session as needed. Sometimes, the leader uses the "freeze" command as an opportunity to direct participants to reflect on the activity.

Example: The group has lost focus and is overactive; they laugh, talk, interrupt each other, and step outside the circle's bounds. The container is becoming compromised. The leader calls "Freeze!" and directs the group to stop action for a few seconds until their energy calms. The activity resumes only once the leader feels the group is ready to continue or they introduce a less activating activity. The leader may do this several times until the group is back on track.

Focus Command

"Focus" is an excellent command to redirect participants back to an activity. The command is called out to the entire group, so no one feels called out or put on the spot. This directive is highly effective for individuals with hyperactivity or impulse control issues.

Example: The leader sees that the group has lost focus, and their energy is running amuck; their behavior is beginning to get out of control. The leader yells: "Freeze!" Pointing to the ceiling, they say, "Focus on the ceiling!" and participants look up. Then, pointing toward the door, they say, "Focus on the door." Finally, the leader says, "Focus on me." Everyone in the group is now focused on the leader. The activity resumes, or a new one is introduced.

Center Command

"Center" is called for when you want students to feel a sense of their physical boundaries and prepare themselves for the next activity. It is good for grounding. Students should be asked to find a centered place in their bodies, with their arms at their sides and their legs slightly apart. They can take a few deep breaths and relax, paying attention to the silence.

Example: If you notice that the class is losing focus or becoming chaotic, you can call "Center," asking them to place their feet firmly on the ground to feel their bodies centered and grounded.

The Three Levels of Theater Games

ENACT's developmental theater games, like all of ENACT's activities, are designed for emotional safety. They are categorized into three levels to build on the participants' strengths, heighten self-esteem, and encourage risk-taking. Each level is meant to increase in difficulty based on the group's feeling of safety, and each level requires increased risk-taking.

Facilitators often take a moment just after a game to reflect on the experience to help participants integrate their learning. Participants are celebrated for success, built into the process, with validating statements and applause from the group after each activity.

The three levels are as follows:

- *Level 1: Unison (all group members participate). This is the safest level and the lowest risk.*

    Unison games foster group cohesion and safety. In a unison game, no one is put on the spot because everyone participates in the activity together. Participants imitate the leader simultaneously, so no one feels alone. The exercises help participants feel safe and secure within a group experience.

    There are many theater game applications of unison games. They can be used as a healing ritual with rhythm and dance movements. For example, a leader may clap out a rhythm that increases complexity, and the group imitates. They can be used to introduce self-regulation skills such as breathing or counting to 10.

- *Level 2: Interpersonal (two-person interaction). Intermediate level of safety and risk.*

    Interpersonal games require a little more risk-taking than unison games because participants are invited to interact with one another.

They should only be introduced once a feeling of trust has been established within the group. These games offer less emotional safety than unison games because participants often work in pairs, building interpersonal communication, fostering trust, and promoting empathy.

- *Level 3: Individual (a participant acting alone). Highest level of emotional risk.*

Individual activities require the highest degree of risk-taking. They should only be introduced when substantial safety and trust have been built so the individual feels supported for taking risks by working individually in front of the group. If readiness level and feeling of support are assumed, individuals are called upon voluntarily to perform an exercise as their peers witness them in a supportive manner. While this activity is challenging to some individuals, others love the attention and are more than willing to jump in.

Below are several ENACT games. Many of these are based on the work of Viola Spolin,[4] the originator of theater games, but have been adjusted for therapeutic purposes.

Sample Games: Unison, Interpersonal, and Individual

Unison

- **Freeze, focus, center**. *This exercise helps teens to redirect behavior.*

These commands help the group return to a neutral stance, especially if the group is getting chaotic. I always say, "When in doubt, return to unison." Let's say you are in the middle of an activity and notice that the group is starting to lose focus and could quickly turn chaotic. Call out one of the basic directives introduced earlier in this chapter, such as "Freeze!" The students know to stand in place. You might then point to the ceiling and say, "Focus on the ceiling." Then, point to the floor and say, "Focus on the floor." You can also call, "Center." Finally, point to yourself and say, "Focus on me!" Once the students focus on you, you can return to your previous activity.

- **Exaggerated attitudes**. *This exercise helps adolescents become conscious of their attitudes.*

The facilitator asks participants to express a big attitude, like an aggressive pose with an angry facial expression and arms poised for a fight, and then directs them to drop the pose as well as their defenses. This is one of my favorite exercises because it always engages youth immediately, especially those with strong defenses. Once they are in a pose with a big attitude, have them exaggerate it and then even more. They usually find this very amusing. Next, they are asked to change their attitude and relax their bodies and breathe. This exercise makes them aware of their attitudes, allowing them to temporarily let go of their defended postures and gestures.

- **Emotion statues.** *This exercise helps youth identify emotions.*

    The facilitator asks participants to embody an emotion and create a statue. The facilitator will call out an emotion such as "angry" or "frustrated," and the participants will create a statue with that pose. The facilitator can go around the room and tap a participant on the shoulder, asking them about the emotion. For example, they will tap a participant with an angry pose and ask, "Why are you angry?" The student will respond. It is very interesting and also telling to hear the students' responses. It can give you a good idea of what is on their minds.

- **Slow motion, fast motion.** *This exercise helps participants deal with symptoms of hypoarousal and hyperactivity. The goal is for them to become aware of their physical responses.*

    The facilitator directs the group to walk in slow motion and then speed up until they are moving very fast. They then slow down to an eventual stop. They are asked to reflect on the experience. Did they like moving quickly or slowly? Was one easier than the other?

- **Shake, jump, calm.** *This is a great activity for working with hyperarousal or hyperactivity and calming the body and mind.*

    The group shakes their bodies, jumps up and down, and slowly becomes centered and relaxed. They are asked to become aware of their breath as they feel grounded in the earth. They are asked to reflect on the experience, noticing what happens with their bodies and minds as they become calm and grounded.

Interpersonal

- **Yes/No** *(Used for expression and communication.)*

    In pairs, teens face each other and designate a person "A" and a person "B." They begin the exercise with person A saying "yes" and person B responding with "no." They switch roles so they each have the opportunity to say "yes" or "no." Next, the audience calls out different emotions, like "happy" or "angry," and the partners once again alternate, with person A saying "yes" with that emotion and person B saying "no" with the same emotion. **Note:** You can provide extra safety by having participants by starting the exercise back-to-back; this will prepare them for eventually turning around and continuing face-to-face.

- **Name the feeling**. *Good for learning about emotions.*

    In pairs, one person demonstrates an emotion by expressing it in their face and in their body, and their partner guesses the feeling. If the person identifies the emotion correctly, they switch roles; if not, the first person continues to guess until they are correct.

Interpersonal/Unison

- **The ripple**. *Promotes creativity, boundaries, and relationships.*

    This game takes place in a circle. Someone creates a movement and then "passes it on" to the person beside them. That person repeats the movement, changes it, then passes it to the next person, and so on.

- **Change the object**. *Inspires creativity, promotes boundaries.*

    Someone creates an imaginary object out of mythical clay and passes it to the person beside them, who changes it and passes it on.

- **Zip zap zop**. *Good for spontaneity.*

    Students are asked to say the word *zip*, followed by *zap*, followed by *zop*. They point to a student in the circle who must say the next word. Student A says *zip*, and they point to another student who says *zap*, and they point to another student who says *zop*. The pace should increase, making the game increasingly more challenging.

- **21**. *Good for team building.*

    In a circle, participants are asked to count to 21. The challenge is that each number must be in order and called out one at a time. If two people say a number at the same time, the game goes back to the beginning and they start all over again. This often takes a few rounds as teens experiment with giving cues to each other before they jump in.

Individual

- **Guess what I am feeling**. *Teaches leadership, empathy, and emotion recognition.*

    One participant stands in the center of the circle and acts out an emotion, making it bigger and smaller until the group guesses what it is. Once a group member figures it out, they enter the circle, starting with that emotion and changing it to another. The group guesses. It continues for all interested in stepping in.

- **Speakeasy**. *Encourages spontaneity.*

    Participants are given a topic to discuss, such as friendships. One participant after another volunteers to speak on the subject for 30 seconds, as fast as they can.

Sample Games: Variations and Combinations

As we saw above in the examples of Interpersonal/Unison games, some exercises incorporate more than one level within the same session. There are other games, like those below, that can be adapted to work solely at one level or another. While the levels may build on each other, it is up to you whether you want to progress from a less intense to a more intense level or move back to a less intense level. Vary the order based on the group's needs, competence levels, and in-the-moment responses.

Clap and Stomp

There are many variations of this game and reasons to use them. They are particularly good in chaotic classrooms to help teens focus and for kids who have impulse-control problems.

- *Unison:* The leader claps, stomps, or otherwise pounds out a rhythm. The group repeats the rhythm. The leader continues by making the rhythm as complicated as the group can follow. An ambitious leader may combine claps and stomps.
- *Interpersonal:* Break participants into pairs and follow the instructions above, with one as leader and one as follower. Then the participants switch roles.
- *Individual/Interpersonal:* A teen in your group may want to lead the others. Go for it. The teen provides the rhythm, and the group echoes it.

Sound Orchestra

One participant acts as the orchestra conductor, leading the group to play instruments and directing them in volume. This promotes leadership, self-esteem, and decision-making, control, and regulation.

- *Unison:* The leader acts as "the conductor." They ask everyone to pick up an imaginary instrument, whatever they like (it doesn't matter if several students play the same instrument). You can ask them to "play" their instrument without sound. Then, you add sound. They follow no particular song but just imitate the instrument's sound in whatever melody or rhythm they prefer.

Next, the conductor "conducts," instructing the participants to play louder or softer, faster or slower, to stop or start. You get the idea.

- *Individual/Unison:* If the students are ready for this, the conductor calls on individuals to play a solo. First, the conductor calls "freeze" to the group, then points to an individual and calls out, "Solo!" The individual does their piece, the conductor motions for the soloist to stop, then motions for the rest of the group to join back in.

Invite a student to become the conductor as a variation on Individual/Unison for this game. Remember to "pass the baton."

Emotion Gibberish

This exercise is similar to the Sound Orchestra, but the participants speak in gibberish instead of playing instruments. This fun game is excellent for spontaneity and releasing suppressed emotions.

- *Unison:* The leader states an emotion, such as happiness, sadness, or frustration, then speaks in gibberish in a way that reflects the stated emotion. The leader has the group respond, both in gibberish and with their bodies, all together, exhibiting the same emotion. (This will sound chaotic.)
- *Individual/Unison:* The leader calls on a student to lead the group. The game is carried out as above. The leader can call on additional students in sequence.
- *Interpersonal:* Two participants do an improvised scene with gibberish, a made-up language of sounds instead of words. The group tells them who and where they are going to be, such as friends at a party or a mother and a daughter. A participant is chosen from the group to call out emotions that the players enact through their gibberish. Once this is successful, the players can decide upon their own emotions.

Mirror Game

Participants mirror each other's facial expressions, movements, and sounds. This is a great exercise to elicit empathy and help with emotional expression.

- *Unison:* The leader creates various gestures, such as raising a hand, turning their body, and assuming the prayer position. The entire group mirrors the leader's facial expressions and movements. Next, the leader adds sounds, perhaps open vowel sounds or any sort of sound, really. The group imitates.

- *Individual/Unison:* A participant can lead the exercise once the group has developed trust. The participant goes through the steps outlined above.
- *Interpersonal* Two participants mirror each other's movements and sounds. The goal is to encourage empathy through synchronization. This exercise promotes relationships and empathy.

Note: *You may also want to try theater games to address specific emotions, behavior, and unhealed trauma symptoms.* Be aware that some of these are more advanced emotional support techniques that should only be used by experienced youth workers and professionals with mental health training. You can find these games and exercises in Appendix 1.

After the participants in your session have warmed up with theater games, you are ready to proceed with the main activity: scene work.

Notes

1 ENACT program evaluation Rob Horowitz, New York Center for Arts Education Research (2011).
2 Feldman, *Current Approaches in Drama Therapy*, 304.
3 Emunah, *Acting for Real*, 73.
4 Spolin, *Improvisation for the Theater.*

Chapter 8

Phase II: The Main Activity (Scene Work)

Felicia and her classmates scrambled to evacuate a school across from the World Trade Center on September 11, 2001. Stifling smoke, screaming voices, injured bodies—these young people's world had become unhinged within minutes.

The shock of desolation and death that followed the 9/11 attacks on the World Trade Center impacted people from around the world. This was not just individual trauma, it was **collective trauma**, a shared experience of witnessing a traumatic event.

The horrific events of that day traumatized many of these teenagers into silence and retreat. They would not speak to counselors. They felt exploited by reporters. Felicia, a 16-year-old Latinx girl who, according to her file, had "a severe behavioral problem" and who, according to her principal, is usually effervescent, "now will not talk to anybody," the principal said. Felicia had been the target of many reporters who wanted to ask her questions about the day they evacuated the school. "Now she has become withdrawn and keeps to herself," the principal told me.

A week later, ENACT was called into the school to try to help not only Felicia but an entire group of teenagers work through their trauma. This group was also identified as having behavioral problems and notoriously chronic absentee records. We needed to be careful in our approach, using just the right amount of distance to create emotional safety. We could not move too directly with our work, or we could send the teens back into trauma and retreat. We would have to use our time-tested distancing tool and the scene-work method for the whole group.

DOI: 10.4324/9781003415022-11

In this chapter, you will learn how to create an ENACT scene that allows enough safety to prepare participants to discuss difficult and painful feelings—even feelings as searing as those experienced by teens living near the 9/11 attacks. (For the rest of this case history, see the end of this chapter.) You will know if and how your scenario met the goal of creating the right degree of safety by the level of response from the participants. How to do so will be covered in detail over the course of this chapter.

The ENACT scene work is a means of engaging with teens to address these adaptive and behavioral responses. It provides corrective experiences to release and transform thoughts, feelings, and perceptions at the core of their behavior. The ENACT scene work is the heart of the ENACT Method.

Once a trusting relationship is formed by building a safe environment, the work's subsequent phases help adolescents discover buried feelings and lost parts of themselves to learn new coping skills in an empowered way. The ENACT Method helps them become consciously aware of their self-imposed roles in a journey to discover what lies below—their true self and a newfound voice.

The main part of the ENACT Method is the scene work, which consists of three steps.

Step 1. The Scene Presentation

Actors perform the scene. Ideally, a scene takes up to a minute but can go as long as 3 minutes. It's best to keep it short; the longer you extend the scene, the greater the chance you will lose your audience.

Step 2. Processing and Skill Building

Actors/facilitators help participants process the scene and teach them relevant social and emotional skills—about 20 minutes (variable).

Step 3. The Replay

Participants replay the scene, trying out new skills learned in Step 2 to resolve the conflict introduced in the scene from Step 1. This process takes about 15–20 minutes (variable).

Step 1. The Scene Presentation

The scene is a hook to draw participants into the ENACT process and to safely prepare them for the processing and replay steps. Specific components are built into the performance to create an optimal environment for reflection and connection. Real names are never used.

This section describes the elements of an effective scene (also called a "scenario"), and then a guide for how to create one yourself. But first, here is the basic formula for creating a scene.

The scene is short, usually a minute or so. Two actors engage in a heated conflict. One of the characters reacts very strongly to the other (gets triggered) and "blows up." At the point of most significant conflict, the facilitator (usually one of the actors) yells, "Freeze!" Then the main character, exhibiting the reactive behavior, performs an inner monologue, revealing the core emotions hidden beneath the reactive behavior. Once that is over, the facilitator shouts, "Unfreeze!" A short, dramatic ending follows.

The Elements of Preparing an Effective ENACT Method Scene

There are six key components in designing a workable scenario.

1. **The context:** A relevant situation that the group can resonate with.
2. **Distance**: A person's emotional state in relation to an event or person.
3. **Intentional mirroring:** Creating a specific role that reflects the participant's behavior.
4. **The core emotion:** Identifying the underlying feeling hidden beneath the behavior.
5. **Inner monologues:** Externalization of a character's inner thoughts and feelings.
6. **Unresolved conflict:** A clash between two characters that builds to a heightened, unresolved conflict.

Before presenting a scene, you must design it with the proper **context**. The scene must reflect the participants, their environments, and any relevant issues of concern to the group. You will have already begun this work during the preparation phase. At this point, you will have determined which issues need to be addressed and which skills you want the participants to walk away with.

If your goal is to teach social and emotional skills without doing deeper emotional processing, you could start with a premade scene. Premade scenes can be valuable for teachers, teaching artists, and parents who want to focus mainly on teaching these skills. (You can find premade scene samples in Appendices' "Sample Lesson Plans" section.)

Nonetheless, it is recommended that you tailor the scene for your particular group to the degree possible.

If you are a therapist, you may want to do deeper work to address emotional issues. You may want to address the unconscious thoughts and feelings triggering the character/youth's behavior. In this case, you will spend more time on the processing phase before you teach coping and social and emotional skills.

No matter your background, keep in mind two key concepts when designing a scene that will engage adolescents, move past resistance, and create an environment of willingness to participate in the process. These concepts are **distance** and **defenses**.

Distancing Techniques in Creating a Scene

In his book *Persona and Performance*, Robert Landy, PhD., founding Emeritus Professor of the NYU Program in Drama Therapy, explains *three significant feeling states:* **under-distance, over-distance,** and **aesthetic distance**. He describes the state of being under-distanced as "flooded with feeling." Adolescents who have experienced trauma are often afraid of emotional flooding (feelings that are so overwhelming they seem unmanageable). If it does happen, they feel that their "dam" must be shored up as soon as possible and rebuilt to avoid such flooding from happening again. Teens use their defenses as the dam to keep the feelings from building up and flooding over.

Being over-distanced is the opposite. "Too much control is at work with too little feeling." Landy describes the optimal state as aesthetic distance (ENACT calls it **balanced distance**), which is "an ideal state in which one is able to think feelingly and feel without the fear of being overwhelmed with passion."[1]

- **Under-distance:** An individual who is under-distanced is flooded with emotions. In ENACT role-play, actors play characters who demonstrate a form of under-distance when they reveal their inner emotional state through monologues and other ENACT externalization methods, such as "truth serum" or character interviews.
- **Over-distance:** Over-distance is the opposite of under-distance; a person who is over-distanced is suppressing their emotions and separating themselves from them. This is common in teens who have experienced trauma. In the ENACT role-play, our characters are usually portrayed as over-distanced, exhibiting highly defended behavior. Our teens immediately relate to these characters because they, too,

use their defenses to keep them in a state of over-distance so they do not have to feel overwhelmed with distressing emotions.

- **Aesthetic distance (balanced distance)**: This term expresses the midpoint between over-distance and under-distance. It is in this state where cognition and emotion are balanced, allowing for self-reflection and the safe access of feelings.

Over-distancing and under-distancing techniques are used in the ENACT role-play method to help participants find a balance between thoughts and emotions, allowing them the opportunity for emotional connection. Balanced distance is the optimal feeling state which can allow moments of catharsis. Finding balanced distance is an art rather than a science; it will take some trial and error.

It is important to remember that our purpose in using theatrical distance is to allow the participant to safely connect with the emotions that they have worked so hard to push away. This is why we have the additional safety of using actors so that participants can reflect on the behaviors of the actors before they reflect on themselves. We often see participants nodding their heads or laughing in recognition of a situation or how a character behaves. Facilitators are looking for that moment in the scene when a participant says to themselves, "Ah ha, that is me; that is how I feel, too!" It's not just a cognitive connection, but "I feel that." It's an emotional experience. I believe all of us have experienced aesthetic (balanced) distance when watching a play and relating with the characters, or sitting in the safety of a movie theater where you shed a tear for the character who just lost the one they love. It may trigger a memory of when you lost a loved one. You may feel the loss, too, but it is safe because it is not happening directly to you.

With the proper distance, that emotional connection will be made. Without it, it usually will not. So, it is worth taking the time and energy to set up this safe experience for our participants.

Distancing and Defenses: How They Intertwine

When assessing how to create an appropriate degree of distance for a scenario, it is essential to consider the level of the participant's **defenses**.

A defense, as explained previously, is a physical and emotional process used by an individual to avoid painful thoughts, memories, and feelings. Some common defenses include denial, blame, and repression. Many of the teens we worked with, and especially those who had experienced trauma, did not have the tools necessary to express their disturbing feelings. Instead, they turned to defense mechanisms to protect themselves. Unfortunately these did not always serve them well and often got them into trouble.

The goal of the ENACT work is to create a safe environment in our games and scene work through the use of balanced distance. Here, participants can feel safe to reflect on their thoughts and feelings without feeling overwhelmed.

Many of the teens ENACT worked with had very strong defenses, which kept them distanced from their emotions. They found a way to protect their vulnerable parts. These defenses often appeared through their self-imposed roles, which, over time, became habituated and stuck. Their defenses kept them "stuck in a role." These defenses may have served them in the short run but failed in the long run, keeping them from connecting with themselves and pushing others away. The goal of the ENACT work is to help restore those essential connections.

Defenses and Distancing in Portraying Characters

Teens see themselves reflected in the characters in a context they can relate to, like a school or park setting. For extra safety when needed, actors portray various behaviors in their roles in an exaggerated way, using humor or big gestures. This allows participants to safely identify with the characters and not feel like the actor is imitating or mocking them, thereby singling them out. This process provides the participants with a mirror to their own behavior, but with enough differentiation to allow them a feeling of safety.

Adolescents with trauma histories are particularly defended because they are protecting themselves against untenable feelings and experiences. When working with highly defended adolescents, actors carefully and playfully **mirror** their defenses by portraying likable, relatable roles with defended behavior. Examples of defended behavior include rigid postures, resistant attitudes, and explosive behavior.

It should be noted that teens who have rigid defenses are already distanced from their emotions, so mirroring their defenses is a way of saying, "I see you and respect your need to defend your emotions. I will keep you safe."

Let's say the protagonist of your scene is a bully who exhibits highly aggressive behavior. The Bully is covering up the vulnerable parts of themselves, and the cover-up manifests in their defensive stance, posture, gestures, attitude, and affect. The Bully is playing a role, and this role is their defense against feeling vulnerable. A good actor will understand this. This knowledge will inform the actor's performance as they take on the physical manifestations of the characters involved. The actor plays the Bully's defensive stance—not as mimicry, but with a carefully determined amount of distance.

In the ENACT role-play process, the participants' behaviors are not judged. Instead, *their defenses are respected for their mission of emotional protection.* It is understood that these defenses block connection and emotional integration, preventing teens from embracing essential aspects of the self, but these defenses—or protections—have been built up for reasons very particular to the individual who exhibits them. Facilitators must, therefore, be careful not to "rip away" these defenses but to join the defended behavior. This is done by **mirroring the behavior** and using it as a first step to transformation.

ENACT actors also portray **emotional triggers** as part of the character's behavior, which is very relatable to teens who have experienced trauma. Triggers are words, gestures, or actions of another that lead to reactive and explosive behavior in the character. This type of behavior happens when defenses become compromised. (For a list of common triggers, see Chapter 3.)

A scenario that has been highly effective with students identified with reactive behavior is the one that began the introduction to this book: A teacher warns an unruly student that they will get kicked out of class unless they sit down. The student refuses, and the teacher touches them on the shoulder, triggering them to explode into aggressive behavior. In this scene, the actor playing the student says, "Who do you think you are, my mother?" and storms out of the classroom. The tap on the shoulder was the trigger that may have unconsciously reminded them of being touched in a way that was threatening to them. This scene always gets an immediate response from students, with heads nodding as if they resonate, leading to a willingness to process the scene.

Externalizing the Core Emotion

To create an effective scenario, facilitators must be aware of the **core emotion** behind the participant's defenses. The reason for working with the core feelings, such as anger or shame, is that the youth can stay stuck in a role if those core feelings are left unaddressed. They continue living in a defensive stance, constraining and preventing their full self from being expressed. For teens with trauma, core emotions are carefully hidden beneath a defense because these feelings are too painful to deal with. Facilitators must be aware of the **core emotion** behind the participant's defenses to create an effective scenario that may lead to transformation.

ENACT uses the term "behavior costume" as a metaphor for defenses/protective behavior. These defenses act like a coat of armor, covering the core emotion resulting from their unmet needs and repressed emotions. In role-play, the actors exhibit defended behavior by taking on behavior costumes.

The chart below may be useful for you as you create characters for your scenarios. By identifying the roles and behaviors of the teens you work with, you can also identify potential underlying needs and core emotions. This chart is a guideline only; you will find your own variations. *Please note that he most common underlying needs are for connection, protection, and safety.*

Role	Behavior Costume (Defense)	Core Feeling	Underlying Need
The Warrior	*I'm brave*	Fear	Safety and protection
The Resistor	*Get away from me*	Defiant	Connection
The Stalker	*I demand your love*	Abandoned	Safety and protection
The Loner	*I am completely self-reliant*	Abandoned	Connection and trust in others
The Survivor	*I am entirely self-reliant*	Helpless	Emotional support
The Independent One	*I'm fine on my own*	Needy	Connection
The Denier	*Nothing bothers me*	Fear	Soothing
The Boss	*I'm in control*	Lack of control	To feel in control
The Apathetic One	*I don't care*	Anxiety	To feel supported
The Star	*I deserve everything*	Unworthy	Respect
The Gangster	*I am respected*	Humiliated	Respect
The Movie Star	*I'm fabulous*	Shame/poor self-image	Validation
The Bully	*You're weak*	Inadequate/powerless	Recognition/Power
The Victim	*I'm unworthy*	Fear	Emotional support
The Loser	*I'm a winner*	Undeserving	Recognition

The goal of the ENACT process, at its deepest level, is to help teens safely release their defenses so they can find new expressions and parts of themselves and so that transformation can occur. What's amazing about this work is that sometimes the transformation is instantaneous!

The ENACT role-play technique aims to help teens unearth repressed core feelings and safely bring them to conscious awareness so that these feelings can be examined, named, and ultimately transformed. This allows the youth the freedom to let go of their defenses.

Developing an ENACT scene to unearth the core feelings beneath the behavior must be built "from the inside out." This means that the practitioner/facilitator first must identify the unspoken core feelings and then develop the defenses around them. For example, let's say the goal is to have a group of students become aware of why people bully. In the case of a bully, their core feelings might be inadequacy or shame. The scene is then constructed around feelings of inadequacy or shame.

Sample Core Feelings

Anger • Shock • Sadness • Fear • Shame • Distress • Frustration • Confusion

The goals of externalizing the core feeling are as follows: First, help participants identify the core feelings of a character. Then, help participants become aware of their own core feelings. This will help participants name and express their own core feelings, allowing them to release their defenses.

Releasing their defenses then allows a greater possibility for positive changes in behavior.

Creating the Inner Monologue *(and Other Techniques for Unearthing the Core Feeling)*

Unearthing the core feeling is the process of bringing repressed feelings to the surface. It is a means of *externalizing the unspoken* (letting the cat out of the bag). It is a safe way for participants to see their own feelings portrayed through someone else's. The **inner monologue** is the principal technique for spurring youth to reveal core feelings. The inner monologue is like a soliloquy, revealing the mind's inner workings. In the ENACT role-play, when the action is stopped at a critical moment (usually the moment of most significant conflict, or **unresolved conflict**), the actor "breaks the fourth wall" by speaking directly to the audience, revealing the characters' inner thoughts and feelings. The goal is to have participants relate to the character's inner world. The actor expresses what the participants cannot express themselves. They externalize the unspoken.

SAMPLE INNER MONOLOGUE

Set up: This is a student-teacher conflict scene. The student is conflicted because they came to class late and didn't do their homework. When the teacher demands the student show them their homework, the student accuses the teacher of picking on them. They have been triggered by the teacher's negative response to them.

The actor playing the student says: *This teacher doesn't understand me. She likes to pick on me in front of the other students to make me feel stupid. I couldn't do my homework last night because my mom asked me to watch my little brother while she worked the night shift. I was late because I was getting them to school. I can't sleep at night because I hear my parents fighting, and I'm afraid my dad will leave. Sometimes I don't want to get out of bed in the morning because I feel sick and don't want to deal with school. I can't pay attention to the work, and I will fail anyway, so what's the point of me even going to school?*

The director unfreezes the other character, and they return directly to the scene.

VARIATIONS ON PRESENTING AN INNER MONOLOGUE

Truth Serum

The facilitator invites a participant to approach the actor and "give them a shot of truth serum." Students then interview the actor to learn what the character is really thinking and feeling. Because of the truth serum, the character "must" respond truthfully.

Interview Questions

This is the same process as truth serum, but in this case, participants go directly to the interview process.

Doubling

An actor or participant stands behind the main character and expresses the character's underlying feelings. The second actor deepens what the first one is saying. For example, if the first actor says, "I don't feel well," the person who is doubling might say, "Actually, I'm sad today because my best friend moved far away."

A How-to for Creating an ENACT Scenario

By now, you may be asking yourself, "How do I do this?"

In every ENACT scene, there is always a conflict between two characters involved in a particular situation. It can be a common conflict, like a sibling fight or another recognizable scenario. The scene is always frozen at the height of the conflict, and an inner monologue reveals the core emotion experienced by the character. When necessary, the scenario can be about an event that triggers intense feelings, like the shock and horror felt by the 9/11 terror attack on the World Trade Center. In this case, a great deal of distance is needed to prevent emotional overwhelm and re-traumatization.

Based on the situation and the participant's potential emotional triggers, scene elements are carefully distanced for emotional safety. The more intense the situation or emotion, the more distant the scene components must be to ensure the participants won't get triggered or feel overwhelmed. However, if the scene is too distant from their experience, the participants won't connect. There is art to creating an ENACT scene!

> ### To create an ENACT scene with theatrical distance:
>
> - The **more intense** a real-life situation with an extreme emotional reaction, the more distance a scene must have.
> - The **less intense** the situation and emotional reaction, the less distanced the scene needs to be to create an emotional connection.

In designing a scene, **always incorporate four scene elements**, or what we call the four W's: *who, what, where, and when.* These are devices that are fundamental to establishing the foundation of a scene in many improvisation styles. If a scene is too close to a participant's experience and feelings, they will feel guarded and closed off to protect against emotional overwhelm. However, if the scene is too distant from the participant's experience, they will feel too emotionally removed to connect. First, identify the core feeling so you know how much distance to create. Then change the particulars of the elements for just the right amount of distance.

Here is an example of one scene handled in three different ways: the first way with *under distance*, the second with *over distance*, and the third—what we're going for—with *balanced distance*.

The issue at hand: the death of a classmate. **The core emotion**: loss. **The aim**: for the teens to connect to their feelings of loss and to find words to acknowledge the death of their friend. **The goal**: for the teens to understand the personal effects of loss and learn skills to cope with their feelings.

Under-Distanced Version (too close for emotional safety)

- **Who**: Two students.
- **What**: They are discussing the death of a friend.
- **Where**: In the school hallway.
- **When**: The day after the incident.

The actors portray teenage students discussing the details of the incident that caused their friend's death. They are both very upset, and one of them becomes overwhelmed and starts to cry. At the end of the scene, during the inquiry phase, the facilitator asks the participants to discuss in detail what they know about their classmate's car accident and to describe how they feel. The class is silent.

This scene has almost no distance for the students to feel safe enough to process their feelings. None of the elements in the scene have been changed, and the participants are asked to describe the experience directly. Lacking emotional distance, the class has shut down. The facilitator urges them to speak despite their resistance, pushing them away even further.

Over-Distanced Version (too far removed for emotional connection)

If we use the same situation and change all the elements but make it so separate from the participants' experience that it is unrelatable, they will not connect emotionally.

- **Who**: Martians from outer space.
- **What**: Two Martians are speaking gibberish and are clearly upset.
- **Where**: Planet Z.
- **When**: 20 years into the future.

This scene may be entertaining and can engage participants, but every element was changed, and it is too far removed from the participants' experience for them to relate to. The characters in the scene are not human and they do not have human feelings. Participants cannot empathize with them. The environment, too, is too far from reality; the group has not been to Planet Z. The timeline is too far in the future for them to relate to.

This scene does not set up conditions that would lead to self-reflection and self-awareness. It would be almost impossible for the facilitator to guide the group to emotionally connect with this scene.

Balanced Distanced Version (allows for safety and emotional connection)

- **Who**: Two friends.
- **What**: They are discussing feeling sad and lonely over a friend who has moved to another city.
- **Where**: In the school hallway.
- **When**: Early afternoon.

This scene needs moderate distance because it could cause intense emotion without it. The core emotion is loss. The "what" element is changed, allowing for enough safety to open the door for connection. Instead of discussing the core feeling of loss due to the death of a friend, they discuss it in a parallel situation, which is a friend moving away.

This scene has just the right amount of distance needed for participants to feel safe enough for them to connect to their feelings of loss. Creating a parallel situation about a friend moving away, while revealing the same core feeling of loss, allows the participants to connect to their feelings of loss and opens up the space to discuss their feelings about the situation.

Extra Distance for Traumatic Experiences

When extremely traumatic experiences occur, or when a group experiences collective trauma, the ENACT method aims to help prepare teens to safely access their feelings, which have likely been pushed out of conscious awareness because they were too hard to feel. The core emotion is still revealed, but in a very different situation with very different characters. All of the elements are changed.

For example, after 9/11, the ENACT program was called into schools to help students process their feelings, because they would not open up to traditional therapists who came the schools. We identified the core feelings of shock and fear and created a scenario with a lot of distance that had nothing directly in common with the attacks on the World Trade Center; to portray this event directly could be retraumatizing. We took the same feelings of shock and fear and created a simple scene about two people bumping into each other at a bus stop and becoming triggered by the other, demonstrating shock and fear. The inner monologue revealed the characters' core feelings. In the processing phase following the scenario, we asked students to identify the characters' feelings and then asked if they ever had these feelings. They answered immediately, saying that they felt that way after the attack on the World Trade Center. (For the full case history, see the end of this chapter.)

Step 2. Processing and Skill Building

The scene has been performed. The facilitator has frozen the scene at the height of the central conflict. Now what?

It's time for the Main Activity's second step, Processing and Skill Building. Facilitators guide participants through self-reflection by asking insightful questions, framing and rephrasing answers for safety as needed. They guide participants to reflect on their thoughts and feelings about the scene and then to reflect on their own experiences.

Like all ENACT activities, this step is designed with emotional distance, bridging from general questions to more personal thoughts, perceptions, and feelings.

The Facilitator's Role

The ENACT facilitator is a compassionate guide, healer, and ally who attunes with the group using non-judgmental feedback. They prompt self-awareness and inspire transformation. They move seamlessly from one ENACT phase to the next. The facilitator regularly validates participants' thoughts and feelings, gently guiding them to reflective experiences that prompt self-discovery.

During a session, the facilitator tunes into the entire group and works with individuals within the group, guiding them to conscious change.

The group is used to contain and witness individual experiences and transformations.

After the scene is presented to the group, the facilitator creates connection by ping-ponging back and forth from the scenario and the actor's portrayal to the group's reflection until the group feels safe enough to discover deeper personal meaning.

There are three phases of inquiry that the facilitator moves through after the scene: the identification phase, the connection phase, and the skill-building phase.

The Identification Phase: Cognition

In the **identification phase**, facilitators ask questions about the scenario to assess whether the group understood what was presented and whether they resonated with the scene. This is handled in a matter-of-fact, nonemotional way. *This is the safest, most distanced phase* because the participants are only asked to use their thinking brains.

Ensuring Identification: Sample Questions

- Does this scene look familiar? Is it realistic?
  This allows the facilitator to see if the group resonated with the scene.
- What would you name this scene?
  This frames the scene for safety.
- What was this scene about? Please recap the scenario.
  This keeps the emotional distance.

Once the facilitator feels confident that the group has resonated with the scene and is hooked into the process, they can move on to the next phase.

The Connection Phase: Emotional

The **connection phase** goes beyond talking about the surface topics. It is used to spur emotional connection. The goal is for participants to align with the scene's characters to reflect on their thoughts and feelings. *It is less distant because participants are invited to be more vulnerable.*

Facilitators use **bridge questions** to help participants connect external observations to internal thoughts and feelings. Bridging uses empathy and non-judgment to prompt individuals to safely connect emotionally to what they have observed, stirring their perceptions, thoughts, and feelings.

Goals of the Connection Phase

- To promote self-reflection.
- To guide participants to connect to their thoughts and feelings safely.
- To help surface repressed emotions.
- To guide participants in identifying social and emotional and coping skills.
- To prepare participants for Step 3: The Replay.

Bridge Questions

- How would you describe the behavior of the character? What was their attitude? Have you seen other people act this way?

Identifying and naming behavior.

- How do you think the character was feeling? Do you know other people who feel this way?

Identifying and naming feelings.

- Do they have the right to feel that way? Everyone has a right to their feelings.

Validates the emotions, demonstrating that you are non-judgmental, so participants feel safe discussing their feelings.

- Can you give me an example of when you or someone you know may have felt this way?

An example demonstrates that the participant understands the situation.

At this point, facilitators help participants transition from observing the character's behavior, thoughts, and feelings to reflecting on their own. Once an emotional connection is made, the facilitator may see nonverbal reactions like shaking their heads in agreement or laughing.

Sometimes comments are verbal, like, "Wow! I feel that way too!" or "That happened to me!" These are common reactions and demonstrate that individuals feel emotionally connected to the scene context and character.

Before we move on to the third phase, skill building, it's important to discuss another aspect of keeping participants safe. The facilitator knows that safety is the number one concern in the ENACT process.

Keeping Participants Safe: Avoiding Disclosure

Facilitators help participants avoid feeling exposed, especially when working with youth with trauma histories. So, how do facilitators ask questions about participants' thoughts and feelings while working to protect them? This can be delicate balancing act, so the facilitator must be sensitive and mindful.

Facilitators rely on two main techniques to guide and protect the participants:

Framing: The facilitator tells participants they will ask questions to see if the participants can relate to the scene. Teens are given the option to write their responses instead of speaking. The facilitator provides the guidelines: Participants can give examples of when they have had similar feelings to those of the character but are strongly discouraged from telling their own story (unless this is a therapeutic setting). Teens should be guided to frame their answers in the first person and only give a sentence or two about the situation. For example, "I feel angry when I can't attend a party."

Validating the feeling and redirecting the response: If a participant delves into a detailed story, saying things like, "I felt hurt when my father did X and then he did X, and then X," etc., the facilitator stops the disclosure immediately and *validates and normalizes the feeling*. For example, "Yes, it can feel hurtful when someone ignores you." Then, they redirect the teen back to the feelings of the character in the scene.

It may seem counterintuitive to ask someone to give an example of a situation in their lives and then redirect them once they share. However, what we are doing is protecting the participants from emotional flooding and regretting that they revealed too much information. We are seeking only evidence that the participant understands the feeling conveyed in the scene. We don't want them to disclose their personal history. Instead, we want to bring the focus back to the scenario, where the participant can safely work out their own feelings through the situation portrayed by the characters.

To recap the main activity so far:

- The scene was performed.
- The facilitator helped the participants process the scene by first ensuring that they identified with it.
- The facilitator then guided the participants in making emotional connections to the material.

The Skill-Building Phase

The next phase is **skill building**. The ENACT Method teaches coping skills and social and emotional skills, and of course, there is an overlap between the two. Once students learn to regulate their emotions, they can better incorporate social and emotional skills. When working with teens with developmental trauma, there is an essential point to keep in mind: Acquiring better coping skills is necessary for them to develop better social/emotional skills, and acquiring better social/emotional skills is necessary for them to develop better coping skills. The two are intertwined.

- *Coping skills* help youth learn to deal with stressful situations and regulate their emotions. These skills are particularly helpful for youth with trauma histories.
- *Social and emotional skills* help youth reduce negative social behavior.

Once again, the facilitators begin this part of the process by asking questions about the scene's conflict point to continue engaging the students. The students are tasked with finding solutions to the conflict to have them learn skills.

Goals of Skill Building

In the ENACT Method, skill building is only introduced once self-awareness is sparked. Without personal connections, the skills will only be cognitive, and our goal is for participants to integrate and instill the material in their minds and bodies.

Social and Emotional Skills

- Self-awareness.
- Self-management.
- Emotion recognition.
- Name feelings.
- Communicate.
- Make productive decisions.
- Resolve conflicts.

Coping Skills/Emotion-Regulation Skills

- Regulate breathing.
- Count to 10 before speaking or acting when upset.
- Use self-talk.
- Ground yourself.
- Show self-compassion.
- Exert mindfulness.
- Identify soothing activities.
- Self-advocate; ask for help.

Sample Skill-Building Questions

- Is the character getting their needs met? *(Helping define needs)*
- What would you recommend the character do to get what they want? *(Looking for communication tools)*
- How can they calm down before they speak? *(Looking for tools for emotion regulation)*
- What could they say? *(Building skills for self-advocating)*
- Would you like to come up here and show us what you mean? *(Getting individuals to practice skills)*

The facilitator repeats some ideas from the group participants and, when possible, writes them on a board or flip chart. The facilitator may also offer additional options.

Once these ideas and skills are agreed upon, participants are invited to come up and try them out by replaying the scene with an actor. This is Step 3 in which participants integrate what they have learned. They can now replay the scene with new solutions and voice unspoken thoughts and feelings, resulting in accomplishment and empowerment.

Step 3. The Replay

All steps lead to this one, the Replay. In this theatrical space, something magical happens. Participants are invited to come up and replay the scene using their newfound skill.

Students who previously presented with poor self-concepts find their voice, name their feelings, and advocate for themselves. Their peers witness them as they step into a new, empowered version of themselves. In this transformative process, *youth find their authentic voice and replace their previous defenses. They discover their authentic selves, letting go of the old roles and habitual behavior they were stuck in*, releasing defenses that are now replaced with conscious communication, and naming denied feelings that kept them from discovering their authentic selves by trying on new roles and releasing others.

Replay Tools

- **Coaching.** The facilitator or actor stands beside the character played by the participant as the participant replays the scene and tries out new skills that were discussed during the processing phase. Let the participant know you are there if they need you. If they get stuck, gently touch their shoulder and whisper some responses to them to help them through the scene as needed.
- **Doubling.** The facilitator or an invited participant stands beside the protagonist in the role-play and voices the deeper, unexpressed feelings.
- **Rewinding the scene.** Stop the scene and call "freeze" if it is going in the wrong direction and rewind it, starting at an identified replay point.
- **Switching roles.** Have participants switch roles to help them step into the other character's emotions and point of view, encouraging empathy.

At the start of the chapter, we began a case history that addressed the collective trauma brought on by the 9/11 attacks. What follows is the rest of that story. You'll see how we used the safety of distance to encourage self-awareness and guide these teens to finally open up about their feelings.

In working with these teens who had been so shut down, we addressed their initial resistance with care, inviting them to join us in our playful theater games. Laughter and fun were much-needed medicine. Within the first few days, a sense of trust was built, enabling us to move into our role-play method. We knew that most of the students in this group were unwilling to discuss the traumatic school evacuation that day; we had to work very carefully and safely to uncover and address the overwhelming emotions they experienced by giving them just the right amount of emotional space to connect. The ENACT scene work was designed for that.

Two skilled teaching artists worked alongside me. Jeannine was a powerful actress, and Sam was an actor/playwright. We brainstormed together to create a scene that would not be too close to their experience but was also not so distant from their experience that they couldn't connect. But first, we needed to pin down the core feeling they were experiencing so we could design the scene around it.

Due to the proximity of the World Trade Center, the school needed to be evacuated. Our students had to escape from what used to be a safe place for them until 9/11. Like many New Yorkers, these students experienced intense feelings of shock and fear, a trauma that rendered them voiceless.

We created a scene parallel to their experience, with different circumstances but the same core feelings of shock and fear. We had to create enough distance in the scene to avoid retraumatizing them. After much deliberation, we decided to change the setting from their school to a bus stop where two strangers meet in an unexpected encounter. We chose a bus stop because it was a neutral space where a conflict could easily unfold.

The principal told us during the initial assessment that there was a growing fear in the school around the Muslim student population, and feelings were being acted out through student conflicts almost every day. She said, "Some students are calling Middle Eastern students terrorists because they heard news reports blaming the world trade bombing on Middle Eastern terrorists." She was deeply concerned about discrimination and asked us to address it. We needed to find a way to incorporate discrimination into the scene. An idea was sparked by creating a conflict between two strangers, one a Muslim woman, and the other a White woman.

The scene unfolds as the White woman anxiously awaits a bus and looks at her watch to check the time. The White woman is caught off guard when the Muslim woman bumps into her while running to catch the same bus.

"You bumped into me," exclaims the White woman. "Why did you do that? Do you want something from me?" Noticing the Muslim woman's hijab, the White woman says, "Where are you from? Get away from me!"

"I'm so sorry; I didn't mean to do that," the Muslim woman says. "I didn't do it on purpose; I was trying to catch the bus."

"Get away from me," says the White woman. "Who are you? Where are you from, and what do you want from me?" As the bus approaches, she says, "I'm calling the police!"

The scene is frozen, and an inner monologue expresses the core feelings of the White woman.

I don't know what this lady wants. Was she sent here to rob me or hurt me or blow up the bus? Should I call for help or call the police? I'm terrified and don't know who this person is; she is not from this neighborhood. Why is she wearing that on her head? She is a Muslim!

Had the ENACT actor-instructors waltzed into the school and pressed the youth to tell their stories, the youth might have emotionally and physiologically re-experienced their suppressed emotions and memories and moved further into trauma and retreat. This is where the magic of the method was needed and succeeded. The scene gave them just the right amount of emotional space, allowing them the opportunity for an unspoken connection, and the processing that followed helped them to find words to express an experience forever imprinted in their memories.

During the processing that followed the scene, the students were guided to discuss the characters' feelings before being asked to reflect on their own. They quickly named the core feelings they observed in the characters. "She was in shock," a student said, referring to the non-Muslim woman. "She was afraid of the woman because she didn't know her." "And she was a Muslim," another student called out. Finally, I asked a bridge question. "Have you ever felt that way?" The room opened up.

"I was scared for my life when we had to evacuate the school because of the bombing."

"Me too! I was in shock!" another student exclaimed. They began to speak about the unspeakable events of that day, describing their escape from the school, running through the smoke and rubble, and finally getting onto a ferry that led them to safety. Their story sparked the idea for a play. A play would be the perfect medium to address the collective trauma through storytelling.

Putting on a play was a great idea for them. "What would you want people to know about your experience?" I asked. "That we got through it," a student replied. The others agreed but clarified that they did not want to perform. Their instinctive reaction made sense because the event was so traumatic that even the distance of the theater was too overwhelming and could reactivate them. They were so raw emotionally that they could not go on stage before strangers and tell their stories. They needed someone else to do it for them.

It was decided that we would use actors as surrogates for them. Our team of actors would perform the play, telling their stories to the public about their experiences that day to open up a larger discussion. The students were excited about the idea and over the next few months would create a theater piece meaningful to all involved. In doing the work, we all had a opportunity to participate in a valuable shared play-making experience.

Through the process, Felicia and her peers told us their stories of that horrific day. Then each student paired off with an EN-ACT actor who would become, in essence, that youth on stage. Each teen selected an actor to play the role representing them. They became the directors, teaching the actors to imitate their voices and recreate their body language just as they would do it. Felica was beginning to open up through the process. Our playwright helped to shape the piece.

The play turned out to be powerful, using vignettes created by each team. One student told an amusing story of how she and her classmates had to run to catch the ferry to Staten Island to safety. "All I could focus on was this pack of M&Ms that I found on the floor. I couldn't focus on anything else." She explained the experience as feeling unreal. Another student talked about his fear of getting trapped in the school and wanting to run. Each story had drama but also included humor, discovered by the students as they recounted their experiences.

The play served as a vehicle to find meaning and purpose from a terrible experience.

Through the process, the group became deeply bonded. The students were gaining more personal insight and discovering lessons they had learned. As the performance date grew closer, their excitement overrode their fear. On the night of the performance, the play, performed by the actors, was witnessed by our student writers and directors sitting in the front row, along with a supportive and engaged audience. When the curtain came down after loud cheers, the students stepped up to the stage, answering questions from a congratulatory audience. Our students moved from being victims to embracing the roles of heroes.

Someone asked Felicia what watching her story performed on stage felt like. This time, Felicia did not withdraw from a stranger's question. She stood up and explained how empowering and uplifting the process was for her, as she wiped away some tears. Weeks earlier, this young woman was frozen and unable to speak. It was the first time she showed emotion in the weeks following 9/11. Through the magic of theater, she was transformed from feeling helpless to feeling heroic.

Author's Notes

- This story demonstrates how storytelling can mobilize and heal, giving teens with trauma the space and distance to make sense of a situation that felt "unreal" to them. Feeling an experience is "unreal" is a description of dissociation, a trauma symptom. There were several instances in which youth described trauma symptoms as they told us their stories. The girl who focused on a pack of M&Ms said her experience felt "unreal." This describes an experience of dissociation.

- Giving youth space and distance from their feelings is essential in volatile or potentially traumatic instances. I encourage readers to listen to youth to determine their emotional needs and engage them in creative activities that indirectly help them express their feelings and, in this case, trauma. The more intense the situation, the more distance needs to be created. In this case, ENACT used the distance of actors voicing the parts to ensure the students' safety.

- Another student described feeling frozen when he thought he would be trapped in school. He then wanted to run. This was a freeze symptom followed by a fight-or-flight symptom.

- Creating a play helped the students understand their experience was real. It gave them purpose as they told their stories.
- Developing the play and witnessing the performance gave meaning to a traumatic experience. Performance and storytelling are great ways to move into action, a healing collective experience.

Note

1 Landy, *Personal and Performance*, 148–149.

Chapter 9

Phase III: The Closure

A high school principal in the Bronx was in a state of panic. She called to tell me that a horrific incident had occurred in the park outside her school involving some of her students.

"Our kids are too terrified to talk about it, and they are not showing up for class," she told me. She explained that it was a very violent incident that involved one of her favorite students. "It will be all over the news tomorrow," she said.

The next day, I entered Ms. Miller's office. She was wiping her eyes from crying and trying to compose herself for our meeting. We sat down, and she told me a shocking story about four of her students: two best friends, one of whom slept with the other's boyfriend, and the other who retaliated by sleeping with the first girl's boyfriend. "It was a love triangle," she said, "that resulted in the bloody stabbing and death of a student."

This was another case of collective trauma that would take a village to transform pain into healing. It was not until the last day and our final activity that an organic closure emerged. As you read the rest of this case history at the end of this chapter, you will see that the closure was not formulaic, but based on the emotions and experiences of the teens and our empathetic attunement.

Generally, a closure is a review and encapsulation of the day's session and a reinforcement of the coping skills and resources the kids have acquired. The ENACT closure activities are beneficial for all youth and particularly significant for those with developmental trauma who have difficulty with emotional regulation. These youth generally have negative self-concepts and difficulty connecting to positive internal and external resources. Closure activities improve self-image, help students learn self-soothing techniques, and strengthen resilience. Additionally, closure activities strengthen group cohesion. Many of these exercises use

DOI: 10.4324/9781003415022-12

guided imagery, stress-reduction exercises, and affirmations. A session should always end with the ritual of a closure activity.

When you get to the closure, there is usually a level of group cohesion and trust. However, remember that some of these exercises may feel silly to the group, so the facilitator needs to gauge the level of trust in the room and choose activities that will feel safe to the group at the current time.

Sample Closure Activities

Note: For all meditation exercises, offer the options of keeping the eyes closed, open, or in a half gaze.

Magic Box

Many creative arts therapists use the Magic Box activity as a symbolic containment of thoughts and feelings. It is a beautiful activity that symbolizes a holding of the material that occurred in the session. The facilitator pulls an imaginary box from the sky and then places the box on the floor in the middle of the circle. Participants are invited to throw unwanted thoughts and feelings into the box and, one by one, pull out a positive emotion they want to take with them. They articulate these actions to the group, and when the participant pulls out a positive emotion and names it, the group repeats that positive assertion. For example, a participant may say, "I throw away my feelings of anxiety and fear," and throw it into the box. They then take out a more positive emotion and bring it from the box to their heart. For example, they may say, "I take the group's positive support with me." The group repeats, "The positive support of the group." Together, they close the imaginary box and raise it back to the sky until they need it again.

Group Hand Squeeze (Promotes Group Cohesion)

Participants stand in a circle and hold hands. Someone squeezes the hand of the person next to them, who then squeezes the hand of the person next to them. The hand squeezes are passed around the circle until they reach the first person who started the game.

One Thing I Learned (Assesses the Level of Group Learning and Builds Connection)

This closure encourages authenticity. In a circle, participants say one thing they learned in the session. For example, someone may say, "One thing I learned is how to name my feelings."

Pass the Pen (This as a Great Exercise to Build Self-Esteem)

A pen is passed around a circle. The facilitator plays some music and stops it from time to time. When the pen lands on a participant they are to say one positive thing about themselves. The music starts and stops again. Each time it stops, whenever the pen lands in the hands of a student, they say something positive about themselves.

Systematic Relaxation Activity

This exercise can take at least 15 minutes, so plan ahead. It can be done sitting in a chair or lying on the floor. Participants are guided to feel each body part, tense the muscles, and then relax them. They are then guided to feel their breath and direct it to any body parts that need release and relaxation.

Guided Safe-Place Meditation

Like the previous exercise, this one takes at least 15 minutes, so leave plenty of time. Participants are invited to sit in their chairs or sit or lie on the floor in a comfortable position. (It's helpful if mats or pillows are in the room.) Some individuals are fine closing their eyes, but those who have experienced trauma or are hypervigilant are invited to keep their eyes open or in a half gaze and to stop the exercise at any time.

The leader speaks in a gentle, rhythmic tone and slowly guides the individuals to imagine a place or time where they felt safe. It could be their room, a grass field, or under a tree. If they can't identify a time when they have felt safe, you can ask them to imagine a place where they might feel safe, inviting them to give it a try. They can raise their hand, and you can briefly sit beside them. Slowly guide them to deepen and slow their breathing and imagine this beautiful space they are in. After the meditation, invite them to check in on their bodies, noticing if they feel more relaxed.

Note: This activity can bring up feelings for individuals, so it is recommended that you let the group know you will stay awhile after the exercise if they want to discuss the experience.

Grounding Skills

Students are guided to feel their feet on the floor, body in the chair, and their breath as it moves through the body. The facilitator asks the group to bring breath to each body part.

Tapping: The Butterfly Hug

Individuals are asked to wrap their arms around themselves, with each hand touching the opposite upper arm or shoulder. They then tap their arms in an alternating rhythm like a butterfly.

Affirmations

This exercise enforces the concept of the authentic self that lies beneath a role they may have created for themselves or that someone else has imposed on them. The affirmations have many variations; choose them based on the day's work. The facilitator leads the affirmation like a call-and-response exercise. The facilitator says the affirmation, and the group repeats.

Empowerment affirmations

- "I am who I am."
- "I accept myself as I am."
- "I am beautiful on the inside and out. It is unfortunate for others if they don't see me that way."
- "I am strong, and I am competent."
- "I am lovable."
- "I belong here. I have the right to be here and stand up for myself."

Self-compassion affirmations

- "I am a unique and special person."
- "I accept myself as I am."
- "I refrain from self-criticism."
- "I am perfect the way that I am."
- "I am loved, and I am loving."

Self-soothing affirmations

- "I am centered in my body."
- "I know I am safe at this moment."
- "I can hear myself breathing." *(take a few breaths)*
- "I feel a warm golden light moving through my body."
- "My arms, legs, and entire body are relaxed."
- "My mind is relaxed."
- "I am cared for by the universe."

Time-Saving Closure

Sometimes, a group runs out of time, but you still want to do a closure. In this case, have the individuals in the group shake the hand of the person next to them and say, "Thank you, good work." Make sure it goes all around the circle and give everyone a round of applause before they leave the room.

Group Ceremony

This is a celebration that takes place at the end of the session series. Bring prepared certificates with everyone's name and create a graduation ceremony. Have each participant accept their certificate as you announce something positive about them or reinforce the learning or transformation they had.

Sample Ceremony

Participants are asked to stand in a line to receive their certificate. Either play music or have the group create music as each participant comes up to receive the award. You may say, "This certificate is for [student's name], who was brave and stood up for themselves." Ask participants if there is something they would like to say or address to the group. Have each participant take a bow while the entire group claps.

The following is the continuation of the case history I call "The Frozen Ones," introduced at the start of this chapter. After learning about this high school's fatal stabbing, which reminded me of the tragic story of Romeo and Juliet, my partner and I knew that this situation would require a specially tailored closure.

The high school principal continued the story. She told me that on a whim, a student slept with her ex-friend's boyfriend. In retaliation, her friend got even with her by sleeping with *her* boyfriend. Rumors spread quickly around the school.

The girls decided to meet the next day after school for a fistfight. Since the school had a zero-tolerance policy for violence, the fight was to take place in the local park, with the entire graduating class invited to attend.

However, the event did not unfold as planned. Instead of just the two girls fighting it out, their boyfriends showed up and began to brawl. They were cheered on by 30 of their classmates.

Suddenly Mario, the protagonist's cousin, a neighborhood gang member, unexpectedly turned up. To everyone's surprise, he pulled out a knife and placed it in the hand of his cousin Juan. Juan was so hyped up from the group's cheering that he grabbed it without thinking and plunged it directly into his rival Jason's chest. His terrified classmates looked on and then scattered, ran, and hid. Nobody tried to help. Jason stumbled out alone into the street and died.

The entire school was in a state of fear and confusion. Principal Miller described students walking around aimlessly, saying that no one would talk about the incident and that some students were not showing up for school. Others, she said, were making jokes. She described some students walking around in a daze. It was clear that the students were experiencing symptoms of trauma that left them unable to process the event.

To address the issue directly, she called in mental health professionals to work specifically with the students who witnessed the event. The students were highly resistant and not interested in their help, she explained. Then she had an idea.

She hoped ENACT could help with our "creative, non-threatening interventions." She was correct in thinking that engaging and indirect approaches would benefit her students because the experience was so traumatic they did not have the capacity to express their feelings directly.

This was a collective trauma that was best addressed by mobilizing the community. My team and I worked rapidly to expand our team to include local advisors, community activists, parents, and therapists. Local politicians were contacted as well. My team worked on designing various applications of ENACT Method theater games and role-play to help the youth connect to their sense of creativity and play and work indirectly with them to process their feelings. Ms. Miller, the principal, was already on top of identifying a parent who was affected by the tragedy of losing his child to gun violence a year earlier. He was now a community activist and offered to come in to speak to the students. Collective trauma takes a village to mobilize change.

We met the students, about 12 of whom were directly impacted by the event, at a small library in a makeshift classroom. They were sitting silently at different tables, working independently. I introduced myself and my partner Alicia, explaining that we were from a theater group brought in to teach acting and have fun, "especially because of what you have just been through." I said. Mistake!

One of the students named Rose looked at me, stretched out her arm, put her hand up like a blockade, and said, "No way are you going to talk about that!"

I immediately realized my mistake by jumping in too quickly before I had built trust with them. I needed an immediate emotional repair. I apologized and assured them we would not speak about it unless they wanted to. We formed a circle and invited the class to join our play space. Rose and her friend Lisa made it clear that they were unwilling to participate and stayed in their chairs talking to each other, but their peers were so engaged in the theater games that they ultimately felt compelled to joined in.

The theater games, such as counting to 21 together and passing the words "zip zap zop" around the circle, followed by role-play, were designed to build group cohesion, which was needed to rebuild connections for students who had lost trust and support in each other. Once group trust was built, we invited them to move their bodies in unison using music and rhythm exercises.

The next goal was to help them become aware of the intense state of hyperarousal they were in when they observed the fight so they could learn to manage the symptoms if and when they needed to. We played physical games to energize and excite them, and slower, more relaxed games to experience the opposite. After each game, we reflected on the physical and emotional effects they had just experienced.

Throughout the games, Rose and her friend remained emotionally protected. They stayed close to each other, frequently whispering back and forth. We later found out that they were close friends with Jason, the boy they witnessed being stabbed to death.

Scene work: Our main goal was to help the students feel safe enough to open up and find words to discuss the horrific experience that happened only a few days earlier. We designed and presented a carefully constructed scene that portrayed a conflict between two young women in a shopping mall quarreling over a guy they both "thought was cute," deciding who would approach him first. Their discussion turned into a quarrel and then a fistfight. With our arms swinging in a pretend fight, my partner Alicia and I heard noises from the students, but we couldn't determine what they were communicating.

They explained that they were participating in the fight as instigators. "We were cheering you on," one said.

"Why?" I asked.

"Because that's what happens when there is a fight." Rose said, "That's how it goes here. People take sides and try to get their side excited to punch the other one out. It's fun."

Suddenly and unexpectedly, Rose and Lisa volunteered to stand beside us during the scene replay, playing the parts of the instigators. They challenged us to fight. "Come on, go get her, you gotta get her," Lisa yelled. "Go, go, go!" The whole class joined in like a chorus, chanting sounds of encouragement.

Suddenly, the scene took an unexpected turn.

Rose moved to stand between us, blocked us from hitting each other, and said, "Don't do it! Calm down! Don't hit her!" Her arms stayed outstretched, keeping us at a distance. She was a barricade. Lisa positioned us to shake hands and apologize to each other.

As the scene ended, I asked, "What just happened?"

"We stopped it, we stopped the fight! We had to before something terrible happened." They sat back down in their seats.

Rose spontaneously began to tell us the dreadful story of the day the incident occurred. "I saw the whole thing. It happened right in front of me!" she said.

"I felt like I couldn't do anything. I was so scared, I froze! When the knife was pulled out, we were in shock! I realized there was a gang member, and I was afraid! I thought he could come after me, so I hid behind a tree nearby and prayed for my life. Other kids did, too. I just stood there behind the tree, and I couldn't move. I wanted to help, but I just couldn't move. We all ran all over the place and hid wherever we could. We were afraid for our lives because the gang might see us and come after us. You see? That's why we didn't do anything. Jason was my friend, he was like a cousin or a brother." She put her head on her desk. "He was my friend, and I couldn't help him."

Tears dropped from her eyes. It was the first time I saw Rose express any emotion.

I looked at Rose and said, "If Jason were watching from above, he would be so proud of how you stopped the fight in our scene today."

On her way out of class, Rose told me how she loved to dance. "I made a dance for him," she said; then she scooted away.

Rose hurried into the class the next day. "I want to do my dance for Jason." She announced. I realized then that these kids had never had closure. They were not told about a funeral, and no one talked to them about the incident. We created a mock funeral service to create closure for the students. We held hands and formed a circle around Rose, who stood in the middle. "I dedicate this dance to you, Jason," she said as she directed Lisa to play a song on her beatbox.

Rose began to dance to the music. It was beautiful. At first, she moved slowly and gracefully to the music with gestures emerging from her heart as if sending him love. Then she spun in circles like a ballerina, finally releasing her pain. The dance ended as Rose knelt on the floor in a prayer position. "I miss you, Jason," she said, with tears in her eyes.

The music stopped. There was silence. One by one, each student stepped into the circle and offered a gesture or last words to their friend Jason. It was the closure they finally received.

The following week, Ms. Miller brought a theater company to perform *Romeo and Juliet* for the entire school.

Author's Notes

This is a case history of collective trauma that revolved around a violent, tragic incident at a public school. While individuals were personally affected by the tragedy, the entire school and community felt the impact of it. Because of its enormity, it was difficult for individuals to process with words. Many students were resistant and avoidant, and others were dissociated.

An advisory team of expert advisors and community members was convened to participate in the school's and the surrounding community's collective healing.

- The students experienced various trauma responses during and after the event. Rose described her freeze response when she couldn't move from behind a tree. The way the principal explained the students wandering the halls sounded like dissociation. The students' intense avoidance and resistance were strong defenses against re-experiencing the trauma.
- Students described their state of hyperarousal as normal: "This is just what happens during a fight." They reported that living in their communities and homes frequently caused them to be in this state.
- Rose demonstrated her resistance to discussing the incident when she held her hand up to me and said, "You better not talk about it." She clearly was protecting her vulnerable feelings. When we

provided the space and distance she needed to feel safe, she finally had a breakthrough connected to her feelings and found the closure she needed.

- When Rose couldn't find the words to express her pain, she danced. This was a beautiful example of feeling through movement, as she embodied her emotions and danced through the pain.
- This story demonstrated the importance of community involvement in dealing with collective trauma. It took a village to mobilize healing. The principal was a strong leader who used her resources. She brought in a parent in the neighborhood who had lost a child to gun violence, spoke to parents and students, and organized community meetings.

Chapter 10

Case History: A Complete ENACT Session

Below is the case history that began in the introduction to this book, with the attention-grabbing scenario of a funny but disruptive student and a frustrated teacher. This case history will cover the entire process of creating an ENACT session, from preparation through the warm-up, the main activity (scene work), and a simple closure.

Troy: The Class Clown

The trauma symptom addressed is fight/flight, an automatic physiological reaction to an event that is perceived as stressful or frightening.

Here are some questions I asked the principal during the assessment to design the plan.

1. How old are the kids?
2. What are the genders and preferred pronouns of the students in the class? What are their ethnicities?
3. Why are they in this particular class, and can you describe their behavior?
4. How many days of school have they missed?
5. What is the surrounding neighborhood like?
6. How well do the students relate to each other and to adults?
7. Can you describe some common school features that students like or dislike?
8. Have there been any issues in the school or community that we should be made aware of?
9. What are your goals for the kids?

DOI: 10.4324/9781003415022-13

My Takeaway and Next Steps

The principal shared with me that most of the kids in this particular class are boys who are Black or Brown, and some are immigrants. There is a lot of bullying in the school, and one or two boys may be in a gang. This is a low-income community. There are drug dealers in the neighborhood, and most kids are from single-parent homes, living without dads; some of the kids' parents may be in prison. Most kids live in the projects, while others are in foster care. They do not respond well to authority.

Considering this information, I selected my actor-teaching partner to reflect the group's culture. Some of my staff grew up in similar neighborhoods, so they could relate to the kids. I worked with actor Charles to create a first-day lesson plan to bypass the students' resistance and gain their trust immediately. But the first day is always the actual assessment day.

Meeting the Class and Creating the Scene

It is our first day with a new group of students. My partner Charles and I need to grab their attention and engage them right away if we're to succeed. We don't yet have a particular student to focus on, as we usually do, but we know that our teacher/student scene usually resonates with almost all the students.

I enter first, playing the role of the teacher. The classroom is in chaos. Only a few students are sitting at their desks. Most are roaming the room, talking, laughing, and throwing paper airplanes. They barely notice me.

Charles, as Troy, The Class Clown, comes galloping in, headphones on, dancing to the music. I portray Mrs. Jones, the agitated teacher, and yell over the kids' voices.

"You are late again, Troy!" I bark at him.

"What did you say?" he shouts.

"Take off your headphones," I say.

"I can't hear you," he yells, "I have my headphones on."

"Take them off!" I yell louder as he removes them.

"Ouch, you are hurting my ears and yelling too loud."

The kids in the audience are watching, and some don't get the joke and need clarification. Others laugh. We have caught their attention!

As you may remember, this is the scenario from the introduction to this book. Troy becomes increasingly more disruptive, and I, as the teacher, get caught up in his drama, growing increasingly more frustrated.

At this point, Troy moves strategically around the room, shoring up the attention he needs from his peers. Moving like a flamenco dancer, he lands in Peter's lap. This gets his attention. Peter is laughing.

"Troy," I say, "did you do your homework?"

"I don't have it. It's at home. Get it? It's homework, so it is at home!"

He laughs. He looks at his peers for validation as they laugh with him.

"That's not funny," I say. "You think you are funny, but you are not!" I move closer to him, and he backs away. I move closer again and put my hand on his shoulder. "Please sit down now!"

This is the trigger that pushes Troy to become emotionally explosive. "Get your hands off me," he says, holding up his fist as if he will hit me. "Who do you think you are, my mother?"

The scene stops at this conflict point. We face the audience in a frozen position.

"Inside!" I call out.

The room is silent. The students are now transfixed. Even Peter raises his head from the desk and watches.

Troy speaks directly to the audience. In an inner monologue, he expresses his unspoken turmoil and core feeling of hopelessness.

She better never touch me again, or I'll hurt her! Who does she think she is, my mother? I don't have my homework. I have no time to do it. My dad is in jail, and my mom works all night, so I have to watch my little brother. I'm late for school? I live an hour and a half away and have to take my little brother to school first. Sometimes, I don't even want to get out of bed in the mornings cause I'm all nervous, just thinking and thinking about everything. Who cares about school anyway? I'm just gonna fail. This teacher better stop picking on me; I'm telling you, I'll mess her up!!

"Unfreeze!" I yell out. Then, "Finish the scene!" With that, as Mrs. Jones, I respond.

"Listen, Troy, you are late every day, you don't do your homework, your mom doesn't answer the letters I send home with you. I don't know what to do anymore, and I don't want to fail you, but you've got to do better."

"Leave me alone," he yells. "You always pick on me and don't do it to anyone else." He puts his headphones on and starts to dance again.

"Troy, stop it now, or I'll have to send you to the principal's office!"

"Go ahead," he yells, "I hate it here anyway, and I hate you too!" He slams out of the classroom.

"Scene," I yell, indicating that the scene has been completed.

"Troy" comes back, now as Charles, and we both take a bow. The students give us thunderous applause. Peter is smiling and clapping as well.

The Principles Employed So Far

1. **Assess ahead of time** by interviewing the principal to prepare for the environment.
2. **Break the behavior patterns** in the classroom with an element of surprise and the art of theater to **engage.**
3. **Create an agreement** to have them sit down by inviting them instead of telling them.
4. **Bypass resistance** by doing a role-play that resonates with their experience so they feel seen and understood.
5. **Externalize the unspoken** by having the character do an inner monologue expressing the group's underlying turmoil and core feelings.

Now that Charles and I have them hooked, I go deeper with the work, guiding them to become aware of their behavior. I begin Step 2: Processing and Skill Building.

"Was this scene realistic?" I ask.

A few hands pop up. I call on an excited student. "Teachers don't understand us. They always pick on us, just like Troy said." Another student: "They have no idea what is happening at home. Troy is having a hard time at home. He doesn't care about school and thinks he's going to fail." *(The scene resonated with the students.)*

A third student jumps in, sharing that he is mainly responsible for caring for his little brother because his pops is in jail and his mom works. "I get that," he says. "My mom works at a hospital on the night shift, and my dad doesn't get out for another year." *(They have made a connection to their own experiences.)*

"Oh," I say, "Yeah, I understand now. That is why he is having a hard time."

"Yeah," the student acknowledges.

"What was going on with his behavior?"

"He was joking around," a student responds.

"He was dancing around and laughing," another chimed in. "He was trying to get attention from his friends and distract the teacher."

"She wasn't being very nice, was she?" I ask.

"No! He wanted to hit her," Peter chimes in.

"What was going on with her, do you think?" A young girl who hasn't spoken yet responds, "She was frustrated."

"Oh," I say, "So they were both frustrated, interesting. Have you seen this kind of behavior before, like in school?" (*This is the bridge question.*)

"Yes!" a student shouts out as others nod in agreement. "I see it all the time in almost every class; someone is always goofing around."

"Has anyone here ever done it? I sometimes goof around when I am nervous." (*I normalized and validated the feeling.*)

"I guess I even do it sometimes myself," says Peter.

"So, what's it about, this behavior?" I ask. "What did he tell us in his inner monologue?"

Three or four hands go up at once. "He is nervous, he can't sleep, he is worried," says one student. Another says, "I think he is unhappy too, and doesn't feel he has a chance."

"Oh, you mean he feels hopeless?" I ask. (*I name the core feeling.*)

"I know I feel that way sometimes. Does anyone else ever feel this way? Maybe a friend or even you?" (*A bridge question.*)

"Yes, of course," they say.

Now, a more profound connection emerges. "What would be an example of someone who feels hopeless?" Hands shoot up.

"Sometimes I feel scared and a little hopeless. I worry about my mother because she gets sick and raises us kids alone. She gets so burned out, working at night, and I have to care for my little brother. I feel like I will never get to go out and have my own time with my friends."

Another hand goes up. "Sometimes people don't want to get out of bed in the morning."

"I understand," I say. "Sometimes feeling hopeless makes you want to stay in bed." (*I bridge it back to the characters in the scene to avoid disclosure.*)

"So, we have a lot of feelings here. Nervous, scared, and most of all hopeless." I write them on the blackboard. But how do you think Troy was coping?" (*Leading to awareness of behavior.*)

"How was he dealing with his feelings?"

"He was covering up how he felt by acting goofy," Peter says.

"Right," I say, "like playing the role of a clown. And he did it well, right? He was a good actor."

"Yeah," he says.

"But was this behavior helping him?" I ask.

"Well, the teacher got mad at him and probably would have kicked him out of class!"

"And how do you think his behavior will help him in the long run, with graduating school and maybe getting a job?" I ask.

They look reflective. "He will probably fail and not graduate," Peter said.

"So, how can we help Troy manage his feelings? Especially the big one, feeling hopeless. They are tough feelings, and you are right that the teacher doesn't understand because she doesn't know. He didn't tell her."

Several hands pop up, but I notice Peter's. I ask Peter to share. "He could tell the teacher he was having a hard time. He could ask for help, but not in front of his friends. Maybe after class."

"That's a great idea," I say, "but is it easy? Troy is all worked up, and I think he needs to calm down his nervous system. Maybe he could take a few deep breaths before he talks to her." Peter nods his head. We all take a breath together.

"Peter," I ask, "Would you be willing to come on and try doing the scene again, telling the teacher how the student feels? Charles will stand behind you if you need help finding the words."

"OK," he says, "I'll do it."

He stands up. I call on a student director to say, "One two three, ready, action," and the scene begins again. Peter does an excellent job playing Troy and starts the scene by clowning around, but when the teacher asks what's happening, he says, "Look, can we talk after class? I'm having a hard time at home, and I need help."

He stops. I tell him to take a deep breath. He does. He continues.

"Oh," I say in the role of the teacher, "thank you so much for telling me. I had no idea! Let's talk after class together to see how I can help or maybe get the school counselor involved, OK?"

"End of the scene!" I yell, "Take a bow!"

Thunderous applause from their classmates! Peter got the recognition he was seeking.

The bell was about to ring, but I always end with a closing ritual.

"Repeat after me: 'Good work.'" *(This is a quick closure exercise. For more on closure, see the previous chapter.)*

"Good work," they repeat.

"Great work," I say. "Great work," they repeat.

"See you next week." "See you next week!" And we all clap.

Author's Notes

- A dramatic scene was created that the participants could relate to.
- They resonated with the scene so we could safely move to the deeper work of self-awareness.
- They identified the protagonist's defended behavior. They named the core feeling underneath.
- They named the role of The Clown and understood that "acting goofy" was a defense.
- They connected to the experience by sharing their own experiences and demonstrating self-awareness.
- They learned some self-regulation tools.
- They practiced the tools of positive communication and learned to self-advocate by asking for help.

Chapter 11

Key Concepts for Parents and Other Caring Individuals

The ENACT approach can be very useful for caring adults outside of a program setting. Parents or other caregivers can apply the concepts to help struggling teens who use challenging behaviors to cope with their underlying emotions.

> **Behaviors You May Recognize**
>
> • Oppositional behavior.
> • Defiance.
> • Reactivity.
> • Resistance.
> • Mood swings.
> • Aggression.
> • Withdrawal.
> • Other defense mechanisms.

If you are a concerned adult who does not have the time or energy to make use of the full ENACT Method, I encourage you to read this chapter in particular. You will learn the foundational concepts that guided the creation of the ENACT Method that served so many adolescents. You can apply these concepts your way (I offer some suggestions). The concepts alone will help you to partner with the teens you love or work with to remove the blocks that keep them from developing meaningful relationships with you. They will also help you offer opportunities for them to thrive.

Much of this book is written for those who work with groups of adolescents who have experienced trauma and have extreme behavior. However, in this chapter, I share my lessons about reaching youth one-on-one, addressing their unstable emotions and unpredictable behavior.

Note: Not all adolescents have trauma; some are coping with mental health problems caused by genetics or other environmental factors.

DOI: 10.4324/9781003415022-14

You may have guessed by now that I believe many behaviors are symptoms of developmental trauma. But even if you believe that developmental trauma does not apply to your adolescents, please do not let that dissuade you from learning from the concepts outlined here. I explained earlier in the book that a study called ACES, conducted with thousands of youth, demonstrates that few of us escape having at least one symptom of early trauma. Learning the concepts below can help you navigate not only your relationships with the teens in your life, but other relationships as well.

Strive for Attunement

You have heard me discuss the concept of attunement throughout this entire book. That's how important I think it is. Emotional attunement is recognizing and responding to someone else's emotional state. It is an empathetic response. Attunement promotes meaningful connections with others on many levels. In my work with students of all ages and abilities, fostering attunement has rarely failed me in building or repairing relationships. Attunement builds trust because the other person feels seen, recognized, and not judged. Attunement is so effective that it is taught to help salespeople build relationships with their clients to win them over and "seal the deal." I have even heard an example of an FBI agent who used attunement (though he may not have called it that) to effectively talk down a distraught criminal from jumping off a building.

People want and need to feel seen, heard, and validated. On a kinesthetic level, attuning to someone sincerely can feel like a form of love and promote healing. You are probably attuning with your adolescent in one way or another already. The following techniques can assist you in this process.

Attunement Techniques

- See beyond behavior and into the other's true nature.
- Release judgment.
- Validate their experience and perspectives. Remind them of the good you see in them.
- Get on the same wavelength; tune into their experience.
- Meet them where they are and begin building trust from there.
- Empathize with their feelings. Let them know you understand how they feel (only if you truly do); otherwise, let them know you are sincerely trying.

Correct Negative Attachment Experiences: "Rupture and Repair"

Your relationship with youth matters whether you are a parent, a family member, a teacher, or another caring adult. Conflicts will happen, and feelings will get hurt; it's part of any relationship. There can be temporary ruptures in relationships, and it's essential to repair them as soon as possible so that a lasting bond is not broken. Children and youth need to know you are there for them despite any rupture and that they matter to you no matter what. For youth with early attachment ruptures with their primary caretakers, any rupture with an adult can feel devastating. If you work with teens, the good news is that you can offer them a corrective attachment experience by acknowledging a mistake or misunderstanding and apologizing for your part in it. It will mean more than you know.

Techniques for Corrective Attachment

- Create a safe emotional and physical space.
- Use validation to attune to individual and group needs.
- Reflect on what you think they are feeling and ask to be corrected if you are wrong.
- Apologize if a relationship has been ruptured. It will go a long way to repairing it.
- Do fun and challenging activities that match their level of development.
- Address their emotional needs without judgment.
- Celebrate their achievements.

Co-Regulation

Co-regulation is an interactive process in which a caring person, usually an adult, helps a young person in distress to regulate their emotions.

This is easier said than done. Most of us become dysregulated occasionally when overwhelmed by stress or flooded with emotions. This is because the thinking part of our brain goes "offline," and the emotional brain takes over. Adolescents have shifting moods, causing emotional reactions and outbursts that can overwhelm them and others around them. When they are dysregulated, their behavior can be aggressive and intimidating. You may feel angry or hurt, especially if caught in the crossfire. Remember that their brain and nervous system respond to external or internal threats. Try not to take it personally; it usually has nothing to do with you. Imagine how uncomfortable or scary it must be for them. Co-regulation means staying grounded and reminding yourself that the way to help them is to stay balanced and not get pulled into the chaos or drama.

The first rule with co-regulation is to apply self-awareness. Try to become aware of your own internal emotional and physical state. If you were to check your heartbeat and pulse, you would likely see it rising quickly. Try to slow it down by breathing or using some internal self-talk. The next step is harder: trying to regulate your nervous system while theirs is out of control. You may need to separate yourself and take a brief time-out while you bring yourself back to stability. Try to remain calm and balanced (at least for now). By osmosis, it may calm them down. If you can validate the young person's feelings, they will feel cared about. (This is where attunement comes in.)

Remember, you may get triggered or have your buttons pushed by things they say and do based on your own history. However, becoming dysregulated will worsen the situation, lead to conflicts, and potentially add more problems. I am not saying avoiding getting caught up in their drama is easy, so don't judge yourself. I can assure you it happens to the best of us.

Co-Regulation Techniques

- Immediately tune into your inner state.
- Breathe.
- Practice mindfulness and remain fully present.
- Stay grounded.
- Validate youth's feelings, but not their behavior.
- Speak in a calm, gentle tone.
- Have a self-care practice, like meditation or prayer.

Help Adolescents in Indirect Ways to Develop Self-Awareness

Adolescents struggling with distressing emotions can find it challenging to become self-aware because to do so means facing thoughts and emotions they are trying to avoid. That's what their behavior is about—that's what their defenses are used for. There are non-threatening ways to help them reflect on their behavior and feelings.

We must be mindful not to "rattle the beehive" when working with highly defended youth. Trying to deal with their feelings directly in this case will backfire. A direct approach feels intrusive and causes resistance, pushing you further away from them. Instead of using a direct approach, find ways to work indirectly with them to help them self-reflect. This allows their protected, vulnerable parts to feel safe and emerge slowly at their pace and readiness level. It can take a long time, but it is a first step toward conscious change. Self-awareness can be sparked by something or someone outside themselves, like a story or a song, with enough emotional distance that it may compel them to self-reflect. The indirect process creates a safe self-connection and can be healing.

Self-Reflection Techniques

- Watch a movie together or discuss a book where the main character deals with similar challenges.
- Suggest writing in a journal as a form of self-reflection.
- Approach a sensitive discussion by discussing a real or imaginary character with similar behaviors or feelings. They may connect the character's feelings or situation to their own.
- Suggest opportunities for expression through drawing, poetry, music, or art.
- If appropriate, discuss your own experiences if they seem similar.

Transform Resistance

Adolescents with or without a history of early trauma can be incredibly resistant if they feel they have something to hide or feel shame around having particular feelings. Understandably, these youth have trouble trusting adults. They will be highly resistant to adults to avoid confrontation with their internal feelings.

Like many caring adults, you may perceive their resistant behavior toward you as a personal offense, but it probably has nothing to do with you. Resistance takes many forms, from emotional distance or opposition to avoidance and denial, or coping mechanisms like playing roles as compensation for their distress. Avoiding feelings can cut off self-connection and ultimately lead to dissociation.

The goal is to help the adolescent relieve suffering by honoring their resistance, step by step and with compassion, to build a connection. You must let them know you are there for them if and when they are ready to connect. Respecting resistance is an essential way of building trust.

Techniques for Addressing Resistance

- Acknowledge the youth's resistance by respecting it and not trying to push through it.
- Invite, don't coerce.
- Be curious, not punitive.
- Back off when needed.
- Join the resistance.
- Do not take it personally!

Respect Their Boundaries and Honor Yours

For some adolescents, maintaining boundaries means survival, especially for those who had early trauma by having their boundaries violated by others. Adolescents coming from institutionalized foster care systems or other institutional settings may have been living in conditions without enough space and proper care for them to feel safe and protected. They may always be hyper-alert and unable to relax. *This understanding is especially important for new, caring foster parents taking these youth into their homes.* These youth may need a lot of physical and emotional space before they can bond, if they can bond at all, based on their histories and early attachment experiences. The hope is that they can eventually feel safe.

For some adolescents, living together in small spaces surrounded by several family members is normal and part of their culture. It can feel comforting. I experienced this during my volunteer work in India, where it was customary for low-income families with many children to live together in small spaces. It is essential to learn about the histories and living conditions affecting the boundaries of the youth you are in a relationship with to develop a trusting relationship with them.

As a parent, teacher, or other caring adult in a relationship with or working with an adolescent, asserting your boundaries is essential. It demonstrates self-respect, which you can model for them. This helps them to understand and respect their own boundaries. This means that if you are running a group, you may have to end a session if established group boundaries are breached, making it impossible to have safe group cohesion. Creating and maintaining boundaries teaches accountability, an essential skill for youth.

Techniques for Defining Boundaries

- Have youth define their comfort level in their physical space, i.e., the room, the space around them, and the proximity between themselves and their peers.
- Be clear about your boundaries by letting them know what is okay with you when they are dysregulated. This means you may need to leave the room and return again. Let them know you care about them, and that you also need to care for yourself. Be consistent in pointing this out.
- Discuss what respect means to them and be aware of cultural differences.
- Once they feel more balanced, you can simply explain the physiology of the thinking and emotional brain and assure them that these episodes will come and go.

Create Opportunities for Belonging

Belonging means being part of a community, and part of something bigger than ourselves. Feeling a sense of belonging means we are not alone. As of this writing, today's youth and adults understand the feeling of isolation from their experience during the COVID lockdown. Many are still paying the price of social isolation. During that period, teens and adults turned to social media as a source of comfort and connection. However, social media does not offer the same satisfaction and comfort as real-life connections.

ENACT workshops are designed to help teens feel part of a supportive community. The ENACT creative container aims to foster community through group activities and goals. ENACT group exercises occur in a circle, representing unity and offering group interaction and peer support opportunities.

For those using the ENACT concepts without a full workshop, look for opportunities for your youth to feel connected by helping them join clubs or after-school activities. This can be a challenge for adolescents who become so attached to their social media connections that they resist real-world connections. Some parents have complained that their teens have become addicted to their computers, which takes on a life of its own, and often, interventions are needed to help them return to in-person group connections.

Techniques to Support a Sense of Belonging

- Encourage or create opportunities for in-person group experiences.
- Help youth establish a community with their peers.
- Encourage group activities that offer teamwork and camaraderie. Examples include sports teams, getting involved in theater, group mural projects, and other forms of teamwork.
- Create a team logo.
- Celebrate group success with certificates or ceremonies.

Share Bottom-Up Experiences (Embodied Approaches)

To be whole, we need to integrate body and mind. Working with the body through movement can release rigid patterns and evoke spontaneity and freedom. Joyful movements and soothing body experiences are healing. We call these "bottom-up experiences." The opposite of a bottom-up experience is a "top-down experience" in which talking, thinking, and cognitive work are the primary forms of processing, such as in talk therapy. Most ENACT exercises are bottom-up experiences. Theater games and role-play are embodied activities designed to create a body/mind connection and spark awareness. These activities can also help regulate the nervous system. ENACT theater game activities begin with embodied activities like movement and rhythm and then call on cognition so participants can reflect on the experience.

Bottom-Up Techniques (Embodied)

- Turn on music and dance with them.
- Engage in experiential and joyful activities like drumming or singing together. Even running outside together. Draw together, sing together, move together.
- Encourage calming activities like breathing or moving slowly.

Help Find Meaning in Challenging Experiences

Some people experience challenging or horrific circumstances and can overcome them by believing the experience has a purpose, offering them something to learn. Perhaps they have hope or faith and believe that finding meaning will help them grow personally or spiritually. Transforming a negative experience into something meaningful helps people process and move through the experience. It is even more powerful when it is a shared experience.

This perspective is very useful following a trauma affecting an entire community, known as a collective trauma. People can benefit enormously by sharing their thoughts and feelings and being witnessed by others. It helps them make sense of the event, know it was real, find meaning, and decide how they will move forward.

Storytelling and theater are perfect vehicles for this. Noted psychologist and collective trauma expert Jack Saul says in his book *Collective Trauma, Collective Healing*, "By rendering an individual experience as part of a collective narrative within a performance space, the theater group creates a safe opportunity to recreate, recollect, relive, and reincorporate the memories of the traumatic experience as understood by both the group itself and the audience."[1]

Meaning-making can be healing. After the 9/11 attacks, a collective experience that many will never forget, ENACT was invited to work in a school that was situated near the World Trade Center. The school community had been deeply impacted. Students were forced to evacuate the school in the wake of terror, and for days and even weeks after, many students stayed home or were shut down and unable to speak about it. ENACT was called in to help students process their emotions. Ultimately, several students joined our theater group, and we collectively created a theater piece that helped them find meaning in their experience. (See the case history in Chapter 8.)

Techniques for Finding Meaning

- Validate the individual or group's feelings, thoughts, and experiences.
- Look for opportunities for self-reflection and point to strengths and bravery.
- Suggest opportunities to express the experience through writing, painting, storytelling, or song.
- Offer opportunities to share the experience with the larger community.
- Point out their inner resilience and how they transform from vulnerability to strength.

Build Resilience

Resilience is the ability to bounce back after a challenging time or a devastating blow and still find the possibility of hope and meaning, believing that it is possible to move forward despite what felt like insurmountable obstacles. Some youth seem able to do this on their own naturally, and for others, having a caring adult who believes in them and works with them to build their strengths and show them their potential helps them build resilience. Being nudged by someone else to push and support you to reach your potential can help build resilience. It might be a music teacher, a baseball coach, or even a caring neighbor who can help youth tap their inner strengths and help them shine.

Resilience-Building Techniques

- Help youth see and develop their inner capabilities.
- Offer youth opportunities to discover new parts of themselves by offering them opportunities to learn to dance, learn an instrument, or play on a sports team.
- Help them build connections with peers by doing a team activity.
- Witness their bravery.
- Celebrate their growth.

In the Appendices, and throughout this book, you will find case studies demonstrating remarkable youth transformations, showing that no adolescent is unreachable with the compassion and persistence of caring adults.

Note

1 Saul, *Collective Trauma, Collective Healing,* 138.

Epilogue

The ENACT Method was initially designed to be conducted with a team and, in the best-case scenario, is implemented by an actor and a mental health practitioner. However, I have good news. Though a two-person team is preferred, one person can implement theater games and still be very effective. I have often delivered them alone as part of a presentation, in a drama therapy group, or incorporated them into someone else's program.

I'd like to address a practical issue that may be a challenge for those of you who want to create ENACT teams and implement the ENACT Method in your school or other setting: *How to find actors*. Below are some of the many resources you might consider.

- Local theater groups in your community.
- Colleges with theater departments.
- Performing arts schools and camps.
- Casting agents (who can vet actors for you).
- Actor databases online such as Backstage and Casting Networks.
- Social media platforms like Facebook, Instagram, and X (where you can spread the word).
- Film festivals and theater festivals.

Team variations can also be effective if you can find a willing participant to enlist in the actor role. Teachers and students (with some coaching) have proven to make strong actors. You have many options!

I also want to share my hopes. I hope that by reading this book, you now understand some of the root causes of adolescent behavior. I hope you will have gleaned how developmental trauma and negative early attachments are often the origins of youth's difficulties, and that it is often these early experiences that cause disastrous effects, resulting in some of

DOI: 10.4324/9781003415022-15

the extreme and reactive behaviors that can make some teens so challenging to reach.

It is also my hope that in addition to learning what is behind teens' behavior, you have taken away practical ideas and techniques for addressing that behavior. The ENACT Method of drama therapy uses therapeutic theater games and role-play techniques to offer teens opportunities to reflect on their behaviors and underlying needs as they learn meaningful coping skills. This opens the door for conscious change.

While the ENACT Method is generally conducted in groups and can be applied in schools, hospitals, youth centers, junior justice programs, foster care settings, and drama therapy groups, it can also reach beyond the classroom. It can be applied in communities, especially where a collective trauma, such as a neighborhood shooting, has occurred. Therapists can use it in clinical settings. Since the approach is creative, embodied, and active, it can be integrated into more traditional therapeutic approaches. For example, therapists who use talk therapy may find it useful to do a theater game or brief role-play to help clients embody their feelings or empathize with others. In this way, they integrate the body and the mind.

The ENACT Method can also be helpful to *you*. While this book examines how and why youth get stuck in a role and how to help free them from their limited perceptions of themselves, we all, at times, create personas for ourselves in various situations. Social settings such as school, the office, and even the home can cause us to compromise our authentic selves, taking on a role to please others or hiding emotions too raw to reveal even to ourselves. It may be useful to become conscious of the roles we play to allow us to expand on those roles that serve a positive purpose, choose new roles when useful to do so, or focus on core feelings to remind us of who we truly are.

Some of the coping skills described in this book can be used not only by teens but by adults. There are times we could all use a little emotion regulation. Exploring our roles and ultimately working to uncover the hidden parts of ourselves can be liberating and transformative. Honoring the vulnerable and/or dormant parts of ourselves will deepen our capacity for empathy and elevate relationships with others.

This brings me to the hope underlying all the others: I believe that in understanding the roots of teenage behavior, you will gain greater compassion for teens while learning new tools for working with them.

Our adolescents made remarkable breakthroughs and overcame enormous obstacles despite their challenging circumstances. I hope the case histories I've presented, about "unreachable" teens who had profound transformations through this work, open the hearts and minds of all caring individuals reading this book.

References

American Academy of Child and Adolescent Psychiatry. Suicide in children and teens, 2024. Accessed July 27, 2024, at: https://www.aacap.org/AACAP/Families_and_Youth/Facts_for_Families/FFF-Guide/Teen-Suicide-010.aspx

Blaustein, Margaret E., and Kristine M. Kinniburgh. *Treating Traumatic Stress in Children and Adolescents: How to Foster Resilience through Attachment, Self-Regulation, and Competency*. New York: Guilford Press, 2010.

Crittenden, Patricia M. Maltreated infants: Vulnerability and resilience. *Journal of Child Psychology and Psychiatry*. 1985;26(1):85–96.

Egeland, Byron, and L. A. Sroufe. Attachment and early maltreatment. *Child Development*. 1981;52(1):44–52. https://doi.org/10.2307/1129213

Emunah, Renée. *Acting for Real: Drama Therapy Process, Technique, and Performance*. New York: Routledge, 1994.

Erksine, Richard G. Attunement and involvement: Therapeutic responses to relational needs. *International Journal of Psychotherapy*. 1998;3(3):235–244.

Feldman, Diana, Fara S. Jones, and Emilie Ward. The ENACT Method of employing drama therapy in schools. In D.R. Johnson and R. Emunah (Eds.), *Current Approaches in Drama Therapy*, 2nd ed. Springfield, IL: Charles C. Thomas, 2010.

Felitti, Vincent J., Robert F. Anda, Dale Nordenberg, Dale Nordenberg, David F. Williamson, Alison M. Spitz, Valerie Edwards, Mary P. Koss, and James S. Marks. Relationship of childhood abuse and household dysfunction to many of the leading causes of death in adults: The Adverse Childhood Experiences (ACE) Study. *American Journal of Preventive Medicine*. 1998;14(4):245–258.

Fisher, Janina. *The Living Legacy of Trauma Flip Chart*, Eau Claire WI: PESI Publishing, 2022.

Fisher, Sebern F. *Neurofeedback in the Treatment of Developmental Trauma: Calming the Fear-Driven Brain*. New York: W.W. Norton & Company, 2014.

Horowitz, Rob. *Process and Outcomes*. New York: Columbia University, 2011.

Journal of American Academy of Child and Adolescent Psychiatry in journal 10, updated May 2024. Suicide in Children and Teens. Accessed July 27, 2024, at: https://www.aacap.org/AACAP/Families_and_Youth/Facts_for_Families/FFF-Guide/Teen-Suicide-010.aspx

Landy, Robert J. *Persona and Performance: The Meaning of Role in Drama, Therapy, and Everyday Life*. New York: Guilford Press, 1993.

Levine, Peter A., and Ann Frederick. *Waking the Tiger: Healing Trauma*. Berkeley: North Atlantic Books, 1997.

Katembu, Stephen, Anoushiravan Zahedi, and Werner Sommer. Childhood trauma and violent behavior in adolescents are differentially related to cognitive-emotional deficits. *Frontiers in Public Health*. 2023;11:1001132. https://doi.org/10.3389/fpubh.2023.1001132

Main, Mary, and Judith Solomon. Discovery of a new, insecure-disorganized/disoriented attachment pattern. In M. Yogman and T. B. Brazelton (Eds.), *Affective Development in Infancy*. Norwood, NJ: Ablex, 1986.

Malchiodi, Cathy A. *Trauma and Expressive Arts Therapy: Brain, Body, and Imagination in the Healing Process*. New York: Guilford Press, 2020.

Maté, Gabor, and Daniel Maté. *The Myth of Normal: Trauma, Illness, and Healing in a Toxic Culture*. New York: Penguin Random House, 2022.

Nakazawa, Donna J. *Childhood Disrupted: How Your Biography Becomes Your Biology, and How You Can Heal*. New York: Atria Books, 2016.

National Center for Education Statistics. The condition of education 2024 (Chapter 2). Accessed July 27, 2025 at: https://nces.ed.gov/programs/coe/indicator/a10/bullying-electronic-bullying#:~:text=In%202019%2C%20about%2022%20percent,during%20the%20previous%2012%20months

Neufeld, Gordon, and Gabor Maté. *Hold On to Your Kids: Why Parents Need to Matter More than Peers*. New York: Ballantine Books Trade Paperbacks, 2014.

Ogden, Pat, Kekuni Minton, and Clare Pain. *Trauma and the Body: A Sensory Motor Approach to Psychotherapy*. New York: W. W. Norton & Company, 2006.

Pipher, Mary. *Reviving Ophelia: Saving the Selves of Adolescent Girls*. New York: Random House, 1994.

Saul, Jack. *Collective Trauma, Collective Healing: Promoting Community Resilience in the Aftermath of Disaster*. New York: Routledge, 2022.

Schneider-Rosen, Karen, Karen G. Braunwald, Vicki Carlson, and Dante Cicchetti. Current perspectives in attachment theory: Illustration from the study of maltreated infants. *Monographs of the Society for Research in Child Development*. 1985;50(1):194–210.

Schwartz, Richard C. *Introduction to Internal Family Systems*. Boulder: Sounds True, 2023.

Siegel, Daniel. *Mindsight: The New Science of Personal Transformation*. New York: Bantam, 2010.

Siegel, Daniel, and Tina P. Bryson. *The Whole-Brain Child: 12 Revolutionary Strategies to Nurture Your Child's Developing Mind*. New York: Bantam, 2012.

Spolin, Viola. *Improvisation for the Theater: A Handbook of Teaching and Directing Techniques*. Berkeley: Northwestern University Press, 1963.

van der Kolk, Bessel. *The Body Keeps the Score: Mind, Brain, and Body in the Transformation of Trauma*. New York: Viking Penguin, 2014.

Weiner, Daniel J. *Rehearsals for Growth: Theater Improvisation for Psychotherapists*. New York: Norton, 1994.

Appendices

Additional Theater Games

For Addressing Emotions, Behavior, and Unhealed Symptoms of Trauma

On the following page is a list of activities and theater games to help teens learn skills to self-regulate, develop a more positive self-image and self-awareness, gain efficiency, and learn essential social and emotional skills. Therapists, teaching artists, teachers, and other youth practitioners are likely to find the following exercises immediately helpful. I have listed these games in a particular order; however, this is not prescriptive.

The key is to pick and choose exercises that fit your group's needs and adjust them as needed. I suggest you use the developmental theater game framework outlined in Chapter 7, which describes how to use the games to meet adolescents where they are and scaffold up or down from there, offering safe and supportive challenges.

Many adolescents, especially those with a history of trauma, have very high levels of resistance; to build trust with them, you must choose exercises that engage them and promote emotional safety. Some activities are specifically designed to help teens address unhealed trauma symptoms as they discover their authentic voice. Games are drawn from the worlds of theater, drama therapy, and other forms of psychotherapy. I have adjusted them to meet specific therapeutic goals and to address specific trauma symptoms.

Many of the games listed here evolved over years of working with youth in hundreds of New York City schools. Some games are based on techniques drawn from Viola Spolin's classic book, *Theater Games for Actors and Children,* and from drama therapist Renée Emunah's significant contribution to the drama therapy field through her book, *Acting For Real.* In the sections addressing unhealed trauma held in the body, I draw upon the work of Pat Ogdon's *Sensorimotor Psychotherapy Method* and Peter Levine's pioneering *Somatic Experiencing* method.

Theater Games

Games are organized to address various symptoms of developmental trauma. On the following pages we will elaborate on each of these theater games.

1. Emotional Awareness.
2. Boundaries.
3. Stress Management.
4. False Self (the role)/Authentic Self.
5. Closures.
6. Defenses.
7. Working with Parts.
8. Trauma Reactions.

1. Emotional Awareness

Goal: To gain awareness of feelings

The Weather Report

Participants will express their emotions indirectly.

Sitting in chairs in a circle, participants are asked to report their "emotional weather," describing their feelings by using the metaphor of a weather report. For example, a participant may report that the weather started stormy and cleared up, and the sun finally came out toward the end of the day. It would mean that they started out having a challenging day that became more positive at the end. The facilitator can try to interpret their meaning or ask the participant to explain. Youth can report the weather as themselves or play the part of a weather forecaster.

Note: This is an excellent opening exercise for building group trust and cohesion when working with a small group. It uses metaphor while providing ample distance.

The Radio DJ Game

Participants will learn to modulate their affect levels (the emotional and behavioral manifestations of emotional experience) and interpret the nonverbal direction of turning the radio up or down as the facilitator instructs.

Adolescents play the role of friends conversing at a party or music club. The facilitator directs them to interact through verbal communication, speaking over imagined loud music and expressing heightened emotions through gesture and sound. Playing the part of a DJ, the facilitator yells, "Freeze," and turns the volume up, down, or off with a wrist turn on an imaginary radio. Participants respond to the directions by lowering or raising their voices and calming their emotions. Once the group accomplishes this, the facilitator selects someone to replace them in the DJ role.

Process the game. Ask participants what raising or lowering their voices was like in response to the DJ's directions. Ask those who played the DJ how that felt.

Note: This game is safe because it is played in unison (see developmental theater games), with everyone working together so that no one feels put on the spot. It can be played at the beginning of a session, demonstrating how the nonverbal command monitors emotional intensity and noise when the "knob" is turned up or down.

Name the Feeling

Participants will learn to recognize and name feelings.

- *Version 1.* An individual is asked to leave the room. The group decides on an emotion and begins nonverbally expressing and exaggerating it. The volunteer is asked to return and identify the group's emotions.
- *Version 2.* An individual is asked to demonstrate a feeling nonverbally using gestures and facial expressions. The group tries to identify and name the emotion. If correct, someone else embodies another feeling using facial expressions and gestures.

Process the game. Some youth have a limited emotional vocabulary. You can spend some time helping them identify and name other emotions.

Note: Version 2 of the game should be played only when group trust is established so no one feels put on the spot.

Orchestra

Participants will express emotions through sound and movement.

- *Version 1: The Orchestra.* The facilitator assumes the role of a conductor. In a circle, participants become members of an orchestra. Each person selects an imaginary instrument to play silently and then with sounds. The group leader, playing the part of the conductor, stands in the circle with an imaginary baton and conducts the group, calling on them to play their instruments in unison, louder, softer, stopping, and starting, and then calling on soloists to play. Once this is accomplished, other participants are invited to be the conductor.

- *Version 2: Emotion Orchestra.* The emotion orchestra has a similar structure, except participants express emotions by playing their instruments in response to an emotion called out by the facilitator.

Process the game. Ask the group how they felt about the experience.

Note: This is an opportunity to embody and name emotions in a contained environment. If participants are uncomfortable as soloists, they can play in pairs. It is very empowering for them to play the part of the conductor.

The Group Mood

Participants will learn to identify and name various moods.

A volunteer is asked to leave the room. The group is invited to gather and confer on a mood or emotion. Together, they exaggerate the mood. The volunteer is asked to return and guess the group's mood. The game should be played for several rounds with various volunteers.

Process the game. Ask the group to reflect on which emotion was easiest or most challenging to read and why. How does this relate to real life?

Note: The group acts as a safe container for spontaneous expression of emotions.

Emotional Statues

Participants will embody an emotion.

Participants move freely around the room, nonverbally expressing a particular emotion or attitude that the facilitator suggests. The facilitator calls, "Freeze." Then, they stop and stand in place like a statue. The facilitator taps on the shoulders of a few participants individually, asking them to unfreeze, name their emotions, and return to their original positions. A few students are then selected to move around the room and observe the remaining students' status.

Process the game. Ask students to reflect on the game, focusing on what their bodies felt like to be frozen in an emotion. What was it like to observe others?

Note: This is an engaging and fun theatrical exercise designed to bring awareness to embodied emotions. If participants feel uncomfortable, encourage them to stop and observe.

Spaces and Places

Participants become aware of and verbalize their current mood.

- *Version 1.* Cards are placed on the floor around the room, each labeled with a different emotion. For example, one card may say "sad," and another might say "angry" or "frustrated." Participants are asked to find the card that represents their mood that day and stand beside it. Once all the adolescents stand beside their cards, they are invited to read aloud what the card says.
- *Version 2.* The same exercise is repeated, but adolescents are asked individually to name and embody the emotion.

Process the exercise. Ask the students if they knew immediately how they felt or if it took time to identify their feelings. They can show this by raising their hands. Depending on the response, if they could not immediately identify their feelings, ask them why it was hard to know how they felt and why.

Note: This exercise is a structure for adolescents to navigate ever-changing moods. By standing on the card, they identify and take ownership of their moods. This is important for youth who have experienced trauma because they often store their emotions in their bodies and are not consciously aware of how they feel.

Safe Spaces

Participants will find spaces where they can feel safe.

- *Version 1.* The facilitator labels cards with peaceful locations, such as a beach, a garden, a lake, or a home and places them on the floor in various spots around the room. Participants are asked to walk over to a spot and stand on it momentarily, imagining themselves in that safe, peaceful space. The facilitator invites them to share something about the space that they liked and how it made them feel.

- *Version 2.* Participants are handed cards and asked to imagine a safe place that is meaningful to them and place it on the floor somewhere in the room. They walk over to the card and stand on it. They are invited to share something special about that place. Before the exercise ends, participants are asked to close their eyes or keep them in half gaze and to focus on their breathing.

Process the game. Ask participants how they felt about the experience and if certain moods were more comfortable for them than others. Give them time to talk about their safe place.

Note: Some teens who have experienced trauma may be unable to think of a safe place. Before the game starts, let them know they can sit back and observe. Explain that not everyone can think of a safe place in the moment.

Group Mirror

Participants will learn to attune with another person or a group.

- *Version 1.* The group stands in a circle, and the facilitator, standing in the center, begins making slow, gentle movements that the others can imitate. The goal is synchronicity, and the rest of the group imitates the movements as closely as possible. Various adolescents are invited to become leaders, and sounds can be added to movements.
- *Version 2.* In a team of two, one person begins a slow-motion movement with a partner imitating; sounds can be added. The goal is to move slowly so their partner can move with them. Switch.

Process the game. Ask the students what it was like to follow another person's movements and whether they preferred to follow or be followed. What did they like about their choice, and why?

Note: This exercise has many versions. For safety purposes, I suggest beginning the game in a group instead of starting in pairs because it is the safest way for adolescents to avoid shame or discomfort, especially for those with histories of trauma. Working in pairs is only recommended if the room has high levels of safety and trust. This game teaches attunement. When done in pairs, it is not unusual to hear laughter. Allow the process to emerge.

Magic Box

Participants will actively let go of uncomfortable feelings and embrace positive ones.

An imaginary box is pulled from the sky and placed on the floor in the middle of the circle. One by one, each participant puts their hand on their heart and says one emotion they want to let go of, like "feeling sad," then throwing it in the box. Everyone in turn repeats the word and the movement. After all participants have had a chance to release an emotion, they are each asked to reach into the box and take out something positive they need for the day, say a keyword like "love," and bring it to their hearts. Finally, the group is asked to release the box into the sky together, knowing it is there when they need it.

Process the game. Ask them what the experience was for them.

Note: This exercise is an excellent closure for instilling positive emotion and creating a feeling of connection in the group.

2. Boundaries

Goal: To gain awareness of personal and interpersonal boundaries

Read My Sign

Participants will explore different ways to signal boundaries.

The facilitator asks the group what it means to set a personal boundary and then expands on the definition. Some ways to describe boundaries are a personal space where a person feels comfortable, and a barrier between one's emotions and the outside world. Setting a personal boundary means ensuring that you don't take unsafe actions and letting others know that you want them to avoid saying things or doing things that make you feel unsafe.

- *Version 1.* The facilitator leads the group through a call-and-response activity using different boundary signals and words, asking them to repeat gestures and words. For example, the facilitator puts their hands up and says, "Stop!" or they shake their wrist and say, "Yield!" The group repeats. The exercise is repeated with only gestures and no words.
- *Version 2.* Using chalk or a piece of tape to make a line on the floor, the facilitator creates two distinct spaces in the room. They ask the students to form two lines; Group A stands on one side of the line, and Group B stands on the other, some distance away. On the count of three, Group B very slowly walks toward the dividing line. Simultaneously, individuals in Group A nonverbally try to prevent the person opposite them in Group B from coming closer and crossing the line by using different signals with hands, face, and body to indicate a stop. When the person on the other side gets a clear and strong message, they stop walking forward and return to their original position. They continue walking forward or over the line if they still need a stronger message but they are not to physically touch one another. The game is then repeated, this time using words to protect their personal space, i.e. "Please step away."

Process the game. Ask participants to discuss their experience with it and whether they liked setting boundaries or following them. Ask them why.

Note: This exercise may be uncomfortable for some teens, especially if they have not had good personal boundaries or respectful limits by others. Let them know they should observe whether they feel comfortable, and pass if they do not.

Yes/No (a variation on the game described earlier)

Participants will practice using words and emotions to express boundaries.

- *Version 1.* Adolescents are asked to stand back-to-back in pairs. On the count of three, Person 1 says "yes," and Person 2 says "no." The facilitator asks them to increase and decrease their volume and exaggerate their emotions to experience the effects of using different affects and intensities.
- *Version 2.* Participants repeat the exercise, but this time, they face each other. The exercise is repeated, allowing participants to experience both statements.

Process the game. Ask participants which statement they liked saying more than the other, and why.

Note: Some participants, if they are introverted, will need some coaxing to increase intensity. Be aware that others may feel overwhelmed by the intensity.

3. Stress Management

Goal: To control and manage levels of stress

Blowing Off Stress

Participants learn the power of their breath.

Before beginning the exercise, tell participants that if they feel weak or dizzy during the exercise, they should sit down immediately. Pause the exercise periodically to check in on how they are doing.

Participants stand in two lines facing each other. On a count of three, people in Line A blow toward the people across from them in Line B to get them to back up, based on the power of their breaths. Line B people move back a few steps in response. As the breaths feel more powerful, they move back. Switch teams. Following the exercise, participants are asked to sit back in their chairs and relax, noticing the quality of their breathing.

Process the game. Ask participants about the experience and how they feel in their bodies. Were they aware of the power of their breath?

Note: This exercise could cause physical symptoms or potentially lead to hyperventilation. Caution is advised to ensure participants do not become weak or dizzy. The facilitator should stop and start occasionally, allowing participants to sit down at any point they are uncomfortable or experience physical symptoms.

Ancient Tree

Participants will feel grounded and centered in their bodies.

The group becomes aware of their bodies, standing with their feet firmly placed on the ground. They find a centered position. Next, with eyes open, closed, or in a partial gaze, they imagine that their feet are the roots of an ancient tree planted deep in the earth, which has survived weather conditions and stood for thousands of years. They are guided to imagine their legs and bodies as tree trunks and their arms as branches reaching toward the sun, sending warm, comforting light through the tree. Ask them to breathe, experiencing what it feels like to feel grounded. After a few minutes, the group slowly returns to their bodies, letting go of the image and feeling themselves return to the room.

Process the game. Ask participants what the experience was like and if it helped them feel more grounded and in their bodies.

Note: This exercise is meant to help participants feel grounded, safe, and protected in their bodies and may be repeated occasionally as needed. Be aware that participants with trauma histories may feel unsafe in their bodies, so always allow them to open their eyes, use a partial gaze, or stop the exercise at any time.

Tension and Relaxation Exercise

Participants will respond to a guided relaxation technique.

Participants sit, stand, or lie on the floor. They are invited to do a body scan as they notice parts of their bodies. They are then guided to clench their fists, holding the tension as tight as possible, then slowly relaxing their fists. They bring their shoulders to their ears, keeping them as tight as possible, and then release. They squeeze their faces together as tight as possible, make a funny face, and then release. If they are comfortable, they can let out a roaring sound. (Adolescents usually laugh during this exercise because it is an emotional release; you can ask them to laugh as loudly as possible.) Finally, the participants are guided to take a deep breath and slowly release the air. They are guided to return to their bodies and come back to being in the room.

Process the game. Ask the youth if they noticed a difference in their bodies before and after the exercise.

Note: Some adolescents who have experienced trauma may feel safer with their eyes open or in a partial gaze.

Butterfly Hug

Participants will learn a self-soothing technique to alleviate anxiety.

Participants cross their arms over their chest, similar to how they would give themselves a hug. Their hands should rest on their arms. Gently and repetitively, they tap their hands on their upper arms. They think of calm or peaceful feelings. The exercise should be soothing and rhythmic.

Process the game. Invite participants to describe how they felt doing the exercise and reflect on how they felt.

Note: Bilateral stimulation activities with positive images can instill positive emotions like peace and safety, and alleviate stress.

4. False Self (the role)/Authentic Self

Goal: Discover the false self and the authentic self

The Hat Game

The game's purpose is for adolescents to consciously try on and take off roles.

Props: Hats and other accessories

Several hats of different sizes, shapes, and colors are placed in the middle of a circle. Other articles of clothing, such as coats, ties, or scarves, are also placed on the floor. Individuals create whatever costume they like from the hats and clothing, then rejoin the circle. The facilitator asks them to create a character and to slowly walk around the circle as they take on that role.

Next, the participants are all invited to attend an imaginary party, where they introduce themselves to one another as their role and are encouraged to converse. After a few minutes, they are directed to put their costumes back in the circle, pick up a new one, and again attend the party, this time in their new role. After a few rounds, costumes are placed back in the circle. The facilitator asks them to shake out their role.

Process the game. Ask the participants why they chose their particular hat and outfit, which one they felt most comfortable in, and if that role reminded them of parts of themselves that they want to express or deny. Ask them what it felt like to return to themselves.

Note: Some teens may realize that these roles are unrealized parts of themselves. In this case, they should be encouraged to embrace these parts of themselves.

I Look Like I Am, But I Really Am

Participants reflect on who they are.

Youth are asked to write five sentences on paper, each one with the words "I look like I am [blank], but I really am [blank]," and fill in the blanks. No names should appear on the papers. The youth pass around the papers and read each other's statements.

Process the game: Ask questions such as, "What was it like to see what others wrote on paper?" "Were their statements similar or different from yours?" Break students into pairs of two to discuss what each has written.

Note: This game demonstrates how common it is to hide how we feel.

Under the Mask

Participants discover their authentic selves.

Participants create a character that may be genuine or made up, i.e., someone they admire from a film or television show or in real life. They can invent them and use their imagination. They step into an imaginary costume, put on an imaginary mask, and embody the role's posture, attitude, and facial expression. They are split into pairs and introduce themselves as that character. Their partner asks them questions about themselves. After a few moments, they switch. After working in pairs, they return to the group, introduce themselves, and take a bow. Next, they remove their imaginary costume and mask and introduce themselves with their own name, and say something positive about themselves. The group claps.

Process the game. Ask why participants picked their character and how it is similar or different from themselves. Discuss why people play roles.

Note: Before participants take part in this exercise, consider having them create real masks using paper, paper mâché, or other materials.

5. Closures

Goal: Installation of inner strengths and positive self-image.

Pass the Pen

Participants see positive aspects of themselves.

Music is played as adolescents pass a pen around the circle. The facilitator abruptly stops the music at random points. Whenever the music stops, the person holding the pen says something positive about themselves. Everyone in the circle gets a chance, and several rounds can occur.

Note: Some teens, especially those with developmental trauma, may find it hard to acknowledge their positive aspects. If they cannot, the facilitator can point out something for them, or they may be invited to pass.

I See You

Teens will take in the good parts of themselves as seen through their peers.

Standing in the circle, adolescents turn to the person next to them and state something positive they can see in them. If they cannot think of anything, they can comment on external factors like their clothes or their smile.

Note: Some teens may be uncomfortable accepting good parts of themselves. Remind them that they can pass, but encourage them to try.

Belonging

Participants will feel connected.

- *Version 1: Hand Squeeze.* Adolescents stand or sit in a circle with their eyes closed, holding hands. The facilitator initiates a gentle hand squeeze on the person next to them. They pass it to the person next to them as soon as they feel it, and it continues around the circle. The facilitator asks them to pick up the pace after the first round and then slow it down again.

- *Version 2: The Imaginary String.* An imaginary golden string is passed around the group to connect everyone to each other. The facilitator asks them to close their eyes and imagine the string going around the circle, starting with the facilitator and moving around the circle to the right. Then, the exercise is repeated, moving the golden string in another direction.

Note: This is a good closure exercise to end a session with a sense of unity and belonging.

Affirmations

Participants instill positive image statements.

The affirmations are a call-and-response exercise. They are great for use at the end of a session. The facilitator says a line and makes an accompanying physical gesture. The group repeats.

Below are a few samples, but you are encouraged to create your own, based on your lesson plan for that day. Additionally, you might ask the youth to add a final word or phrase that relates to any of the affirmations.

Confidence

- I am strong.
- I am confident.
- I have my arms and legs.
- I am a good friend.
- I can stand on my own two feet.
- I trust myself.
- I am brave.

Gratitude

- I am thankful.
- I have friends.
- I have myself.
- I am grateful.

Self-Love

- I like myself.
- I love myself.
- I am kind to myself.
- I am enough.
- I am worthy of love and respect.
- I am special.
- I am enough.

Inner Peace

- I know how to be calm.
- I know how to breathe.
- When I am nervous I can count to 10, exercise, talk to a friend, or listen to music.
- I can find inner peace.

Inner Safety

- Sometimes I feel nervous or afraid. But I can find a place where I feel safe:
  - It may be a person.
  - It may be a special place.
  - It may be a place inside.
- I can find inner safety.

Self-Advocacy

- I ask for help when I need it.
- I allow others to help me.
- Asking for help makes me strong, not weak.
- I allow myself to ask for what I need.
- I deserve to ask for what I need.

The next series of games address symptoms of trauma. It is recommended that a professional with mental health training conduct these activities. *These games should be played only once trust and support have been established with the group. Recommended ages: 16 and up.* The facilitator should use their expertise to vary the games and deepen the discussion based on the group response. Consider telling the participants that they can find a time to speak to you individually if they'd like, or refer them to an appropriate mental health professional if something arises that needs more attention.

6. Defenses

Goal: To understand the purpose of defenses and discover positive coping skills to replace them.

Before embarking on the exercises, the facilitator explains that at times we all have difficult feelings, and sometimes we don't want to deal with them. We use defense mechanisms to protect ourselves from thinking or feeling these difficult emotions, and usually, we are unaware we are using them. Defenses can stop feelings from bothering us, but they also block good feelings and can get in the way of relationships. Defenses are often exhibited by attitudes and behaviors.

Name the Defense

Participants will learn the names of common defenses.

The facilitator does a call-and-response activity in which the participants name and embody the defense, mirroring the facilitator's gestures and words. For example, the facilitator says the word "blame" and points their finger at someone. The group repeats the word blame and makes the same gesture. The facilitator continues the call-and-response, naming various defenses, such as denial, avoidance, and projection. The facilitator writes the defense names on the board or flip chart.

Process the game. Discuss how defenses are common. Review the defenses from the exercise and ask the adolescents to report, with a show of hands, if they know anyone who has used these defenses, including themselves. Ask them what these defenses may look like when they embody them.

Note: Ask the participants if they would like to explore defense mechanisms that they have observed in others. Remind them that no names should be used.

The Attitude Game

Participants will become conscious of how they use attitudes to defend against vulnerable feelings.

Adolescents are invited to put on their biggest, "baddest" attitude. The facilitator encourages them to exaggerate their facial expressions and gestures. The facilitator yells "freeze" to indicate they should hold the pose. After a few seconds, the facilitator taps a few students on their shoulders, asking them to release the position so others can observe them, and then have them return to their attitude pose. Next, they are invited to portray the opposite attitude: open and relaxed. The facilitator guides them to relax the muscles in each part of their body, including their face. After a few seconds, they are asked to shake off the pose and return to neutral positions.

Process the game. Ask the adolescents to reflect on the game, thinking about which pose they preferred, the attitude or the relaxed pose. Discuss the differences between poses. Ask if they felt more comfortable in the attitude or relaxed poses and why.

Note: Some adolescents may say they are more comfortable in the attitude pose than the relaxed pose, especially if they have experienced trauma and are hypervigilant. This is likely because the pose feels protective to them and may be necessary in environments where they are not safe. However, teaching them to become aware of defenses helps them know the difference so they can consciously choose when and where to use them.

Cross the Line

Participants will learn to identify and name common defenses.

The group stands in a line. If there are many participants, they can form two lines. Draw an imaginary line or mark the floor with masking tape. Adolescents are invited to cross the line if they agree with the facilitator's statements. The facilitator makes the following statements, after which the participants follow the instructions.

- Cross the line if you feel you were ever blamed.
- Cross the line if you ever blamed someone.
- Cross the line if someone you know has ever denied something and you knew they were lying.

- Cross the line if you ever denied something.
- Cross the line if you know someone who avoids things by ignoring them or not doing them.
- Cross the line if you tend to deny things.

Process the game. Ask them if they notice how many people have crossed the line, indicating they are not alone. You can deepen the conversation about defenses if indicated.

Note: This game normalizes adolescent defenses and allows participants to become accountable for their behaviors.

I Didn't Do It

Participants will understand the blame and denial defenses.

- *Version 1.* Two parallel lines are formed, and teens face a partner across from them. Group A participants say, "I didn't do it!" Group B responds, saying, "Yes, you did!" This goes back and forth several times, and then the groups switch statements so both can experience saying and responding to the statements. They are directed to exaggerate their behavior. Next, the facilitator calls out different emotions for them to express while repeating the phrases.

Process the game. Ask the students if they prefer being the accuser or the responder. Why? Review the defenses: blame and denial.

Note: This game is fun for adolescents because they commonly exhibit these defenses.

- *Version 2.* Participants are split into partner pairs. The facilitator gives them statements to say, demonstrating the defense, such as "You stole my pen" and "No, I didn't." They switch. If the game is going well, they devise their own statements demonstrating the defenses: blame and denial.

Process the game. Review the purpose of the blame and denial defense. Ask participants why people use defenses and invite them to give examples of situations in which people use the defenses of blame and denial.

Note: Remind the group that the sentences must be general. If students become too activated, stop the games.

Excuses, Excuses

Participants will learn to recognize the avoidance defense and find alternatives.

- *Version 1.* Adolescents are invited to do a mini-scene in pairs. One friend pressures the other friend to come to a party with them. The friend does not want to go, and instead of explaining the reason (they don't feel they have the right outfit), they avoid answering, using various excuses, such as they don't feel well, something suddenly has come up, etc., until the pressuring friend gives up and leaves. They switch roles and repeat the exercise.
- *Version 2.* The role-play is repeated, but the friend drops the defense this time and explains why they don't want to go to the party. Amicably, they work out a solution.

Process the game. Ask participants what defense the friend used to avoid going to the party and why. Discuss the alternative in Version 2.

Note: You can deepen the conversation by asking related questions and having them identify real-life situations where youth use defenses.

The Blame Game

Participants will understand the blame defense and find alternative coping skills.

In pairs, adolescents are directed to use two statements, one laying blame, and the other denying the blame. Partner A says, "You did it!" pointing their finger. Partner B denies it. The facilitator directs them to exaggerate their expressions and raise their volume. They swap roles. The facilitator then asks the pair to develop mini-scenarios. For example, one teen may say "You stole my pen!" while pointing a finger at them. The other denies it saying, "No I didn't, someone else did it."

Process the game. Ask participants which role they prefer, the blamer or the denier. Guide them to reflect on why people blame others and provide examples (without naming names).

Note: The role-play demonstrates how youth use their defenses.

Truth Serum

Participants identify defended behavior and the underlying feelings.

- *Version 1.* A participant is selected to be "the denier." The facilitator secretly tells them to act sad because their friend has moved out of town and to play the opposite feeling to cover up the truth with statements such as "I am fine" or "everything is good." A volunteer is selected from the group to come up and give the denier a shot in the arm of truth serum, which immediately causes them to tell the truth. They reveal the real situation and their real feelings. The game is repeated with other volunteers. The facilitator asks the group for different hidden emotions and statements of denial, which are revealed when a participant is given truth serum.

Process the game. Ask the youth about the experience and discuss why people hide their feelings. They can give examples without naming names.

Note: The group's answers can be revealing.

- *Version 2.* This version starts the same way as the first, but instead of truth serum, when the facilitator says "freeze," the participant uses an inner monologue to voice what is unspoken. Be sure to begin this version by demonstrating an inner monologue so that participants learn how to do it.

Process the game. Ask participants why some people dislike revealing certain feelings. They can give examples, but consider having them answer in the third person to avoid disclosure.

Note: Participants may reveal information about themselves. Be mindful of disclosure.

Positive Protection Toolbox

Participants instill positive coping skills for protective behaviors.

Step 1. Ask participants to name positive ways to protect feelings without avoiding, blaming, or denying them. Ask them what they can do to feel better instead of resorting to defenses. The facilitator writes suggestions on the blackboard or a large piece of paper. If positive coping tools are not identified, suggest the following:

- Walk away.
- Name the feeling with words if they feel safe.
- Count to 10 internally.
- Put an imaginary protective light around them.
- Do the butterfly hug.
- Disengage from a situation.
- Self-advocate.
- Ask for help.

Step 2. Bring out the Magic Box, an exercise referred to earlier. Participants pull a large imaginary protection toolbox from the sky, bring it down, and place it in the middle of the circle. One by one, they name and pull out a positive protection. Once several are pulled from the toolbox, take a few deep breaths together and then release the toolbox back to the sky, knowing it is there when they need it.

Process the game. Review why people use defenses and discuss how they felt using positive tools. Could they use one or more of these positive tools instead of the defense?

Note: This exercise can be challenging since youth are used to using their defenses.

7. Working with Emotional Parts[1]

Goal: To discover the purpose of internal parts

The Interview

Participants will give voice to different emotional parts.

The room is set up with four chairs in front of the room. The other chairs are in a semicircle. Teens volunteer to be the guests on a television panel, and they sit at the front of the room. The facilitator, holding a fake microphone, begins playing the host of a popular television show. They introduce the show, saying, "Today, our esteemed guests have been kind enough to allow us to interview them so we can learn from their expertise. Their names are *Anger, Fear, Shame*, and *Strength*. If we are lucky, we may have other esteemed guests who may join the show later."

Each of the four volunteers chooses one of the "esteemed guests" to play, creating a character who is the human embodiment of that emotion. They portray the character's posture, gestures, and tone. The host asks them questions, such as what colors they like, what kinds of food they eat, and what it is like to get through a day. What makes them happy, what makes them sad, etc. Then, the television audience (other participants) are invited to ask the questions as the imaginary microphone is passed around.

A student playing the role of Anger might say something like, "I see red all the time, and I get very hot. I am always hungry and I like tacos with hot sauce. I always get into fights with people, but I know how to defend myself."

The host invites other guests to select and embody another emotion, such as Confusion or Denial, and join the panel. The television audience will interview them.

Process the game. Explain that we all have different emotional parts within us, and they are all there to help us in some way, even if it doesn't seem that way. The goal is how and if to call up those parts over ourselves. Ask the group how they think emotions protect or assist people.

Angel/Devil

Participants will understand that their emotional parts are willing to communicate with them.

The facilitator explains how emotional parts can both help and hurt them. For example, an angry part may compel someone to respond in a productive way to an injustice, but it can also get them into trouble if they are aggressive. A fearful part may motivate someone to get out of harm's way, but it can also keep them from having new, positive experiences. Once an individual knows what the emotion needs, that part can either help them or they can ask it to step aside.

Three volunteers are invited to come forward. One volunteer is singled out, and the other two participants stand on each side of them. One plays an angel and the other plays the devil. The facilitator calls out an emotion, like anger, and the person in the middle asks what they should do. The angel explains why the emotion is helpful, and the devil explains how the emotion can be used in a negative or destructive way. The person in the middle asks either the angel or the devil to step aside and then explains why they made that choice. Other participants call out additional emotions, and the process with the angel and the devil is repeated.

Process the game. Explain that each emotional part of ourselves serves a purpose and is worthy of respect and compassion, even though we may ask it to step aside in certain situations.

Note: A deeper discussion may be warranted, as some may find it difficult to believe that all their parts are trying to help. In other words, every part, or emotion, believes that it has a job to do. Sometimes it does, but other times, the emotion gets in the way.

Shame Monster

Participants will understand how to recognize and cope with shame.

Adolescents are split into two groups. In the first group, one person takes on a pose representing shame, and others physically connect themselves to the "statue" to create a "shame monster." The other group observes. The statue starts to move, and sounds can be added. Once the monster seems complete, the facilitator yells, "Freeze!" The facilitator asks the monster what it needs to calm down or go away. Then the facilitator turns to the group that is observing and asks for compassionate suggestions, such as "assurance" or "love." Once the group decides, they call out the word, and the facilitator directs the monster to melt into the ground.

Process the game. Discuss shame and why it can feel like an internal monster. Inquire compassionately about why it is so hard to deal with shame. Work on coping skills to manage shame.

Coping Skills for Dealing with Shame

- Positive self-talk.
- Self-acceptance.
- Self-compassion.
- Remembering all the strong positive aspects of the self.

Note: Shame is a common symptom for many youth, especially those with developmental trauma.

8. Trauma Reactions

Goal: To understand trauma responses and find alternative coping skills.

Machine Game

Participants will understand dysregulation (the inability to respond to and manage an emotional state) and learn self-regulation tools.

Using their bodies, adolescents build a machine. One participant begins by becoming one part of a machine. One by one, others come up and interconnect as other machine parts. They move together in repetitive machine-like movements and are invited to add sounds. The machine runs smoothly until the facilitator directs it to speed up faster and faster. Then they are directed to split off in different directions, moving and making sounds randomly, representing the machine going out of control. The facilitator yells, "Freeze!" and the game ends.

Process the game. Ask participants to reflect on the experience. Have them describe what happened to the machine and how they felt playing it. Did their breathing speed up? Did their hearts beat faster? You can explain that this is sometimes called dysregulation or hyperarousal. Has this feeling ever happened to them? What other sensations do people have when they are in this state?

Identify self-regulation skills such as breathing, self-talk, and counting to 10. Ask them to identify other ways to calm their nervous systems. Write regulation tools on the board or flip chart.

Note: Some group participants may not feel comfortable connecting physically with other participants. Offer them the alternative of standing beside a machine part instead of physically connecting.

The Roller Coaster Ride

Participants will understand and manage symptoms of hyperarousal.

The facilitator and one or two participants perform a mini role-play about friends at an amusement park. One friend tries to convince the other to go on the new, extra-long roller coaster ride. Their friend explains that they do not like the physical feeling and do not want to go on the ride. The other friend tries to convince them and describes the physical sensations of a rapid heartbeat, breath, and sweating that happens to their body, describing the excitement as the roller coaster car picks up speed, goes to the top point, and then quickly drops down. One likes the activating feeling, and the other doesn't. They end up in a conflict, and the first friend takes the ride alone.

Process the game. Review the role-play scenario. Discuss the physical sensations that were described. Ask if the group can give examples of other situations in which they or others have felt similar sensations of racing heart, thoughts, or breathing. Ask them if they like or do not like the feeling (note, some students with trauma histories are very used to feeling that way, so they may enjoy it). Once the physical sensations are described, solicit strategies for self-regulation skills to manage the physical symptoms. Write them on the board or a flip chart.

Sample Self-Regulation Skills

- Slow down the breathing.
- Take a few deep, long breaths.
- Count to 10.
- Listen to music.
- Take a walk.
- Speak to a friend.
- Do a butterfly hug.

Note: Be mindful of disclosure.

Rag Doll

Participants will understand and manage the symptoms of hypoarousal.

A participant portrays a rag doll. Other participants are invited to try to get the doll to stand up straight, but it goes limp and falls to the floor. Finally, they try to raise the rag doll from the floor, but it lies there, looking lifeless. Several rounds with different participants can be played.

Process the game. Ask the youth to describe the scenario and what happened with the doll. Tell them it is a metaphor for someone who exhibits extremely low energy and who can't seem to rev up. Let them know that this is called "hypoarousal." See if they can describe symptoms of low energy, including pace, breath, and heartbeat, inquiring if they have ever felt this way or have seen peers in this condition. Solicit suggestions for how to energize if they or someone else feel this way. Write skills for energizing on the board or flip chart.

Tips for Energizing

- Get up and stretch.
- Drink a cold glass of water.
- Find a way to laugh.
- Have a snack.

Note: This game should only be played and processed if the group has developed trust.

Where Are You Now?

Participants will understand dissociation.

The facilitator asks for a volunteer to participate in a short role-play. They prep the student to play the part of a frustrated teacher. The facilitator plays the role of a student who can't focus on the lesson and keeps staring out the window. The teacher tells the student to focus, pay attention, and stop looking out the window. The student tries but cannot focus and returns to staring out the window. The teacher becomes more frustrated until a conflict occurs between them. Finally, the teacher accuses the student of being spaced out and disrespectful, and the student yells, "Leave me alone!" The facilitator, as the student, performs a brief inner monologue explaining that difficult things happen sometimes at home and they just can't deal with it, so it's easier to just "space out."

Process the scene. Ask the group to explain what is happening with the student physically and emotionally in the scenario. Explain why some people get distracted to avoid feelings, and if appropriate, explain dissociation. Continue the discussion at their comfort level. Identify coping skills.

Note: Be mindful of disclosure.

Grounding Exercise

Participants will feel centered and grounded.

As they sit in their chairs, participants are asked to notice their bodies. Are they comfortable or are there parts of their bodies that feel stiff and tight? They relax those parts. They feel the weight of their bodies in their chairs and place their feet firmly on the ground as if they are the roots of a tree in the ground. They are guided to take deep breaths. They can keep their eyes open, closed, or half-gazed. The facilitator leads them through a grounding visualization, asking them to imagine a beam of light passing from the sky down through them to the earth.

Process the exercise: Ask participants to reflect on how they felt before and after the exercise.

Note: Remember to remind students that they can keep their eyes open or in a half-gaze if they are uncomfortable with their eyes closed. They can also pass on the exercise.

Fight/Flight/Collapse

Participants will embody and understand four common trauma symptoms: freeze, fight, flight, and collapse.

The facilitator explains the physiological reactions of freeze, flight, fight, and collapse, which can occur when an individual faces an actual or perceived threat. These reactions are similar to the survival responses to danger by animals in the wild.

The facilitator then demonstrates the trauma responses, explaining each one as a common response to danger for people who have or have faced a severe difficulty or trauma. Then they name each response and hold it in a pose as the group imitates it. For example, the facilitator might yell "fight!" and put their hands up as if in a boxing match. After each pose, they shake it out.

Process the game. Ask participants what the experience felt like for them. Ask them to identify real-life situations where these responses could happen and if they have ever seen anyone show these reactions. If appropriate, you can ask them if they have had any of these responses. Depending on the responses, you can deepen the discussion.

Note: Consider telling the participants that they can find a time to speak to you individually if they'd like, or refer them to an appropriate mental health professional if something arises that needs more attention.

Identify Coping Skills

Coping Skill 1: Self-reassurance. In a non-threatening situation, participants can remind themselves that they are not in danger. Something has upset them or triggered a memory, but they can remind themselves that nothing terrible is happening now.

Coping Skill 2: Observe and notice. Notice your body and breathing. Remind yourself that you are safe and nothing is happening now.

Note: Teens who live in areas where violence is common may be in fear of real danger, and it is important to acknowledge that.

Note

1 These exercises are based on the work of Richard Schwartz, developer of a method called Internal Family Systems.

Additional Case Histories

The following case histories demonstrate how the ENACT Method was used in school classrooms, school hospital programs, special education classes, and alternative school settings. They depict group work focusing on a particular individual within the group. These cases in particular are memorable to me.

Jose: The Powerless One
Underlying Need: Protection

Carlos and I worked in a Bronx classroom with all boys, aged 14–17. They had been tagged with the "acting-out behavior" label. The class consisted primarily of Latinx teens and several new immigrants. We were told that most students lived in local housing projects or government-run foster care systems.

Ms. Stein, the principal, warned us that the class had students who would become so explosive if they got triggered that their classroom teacher was afraid to teach her lessons and couldn't manage their behavior. She needed help. The principal also believed that the class included one or more gang members. My partner Carlos later explained that some gang members in this neighborhood wore red to represent their gang. He revealed that he grew up in a neighborhood nearby.

Carlos was a perfect match for the job because he understood the community and had strong acting skills that could represent the type of reactive behavior that was common here. He also had an affinity for helping kids. On the first day, Carlos took the lead and stood before the class, introducing himself. His commanding presence interrupted their chaos and grabbed their attention immediately.

Once the class was engaged, we jumped into our tried-and-true teacher/student conflict scene. Charles portrayed an aggressive and explosive student, matching the behavior of many of the students the principal described. When the teacher triggered the student by placing a hand on their shoulder and directing them to sit down, Carlos picked up his chair as if to throw it down, almost striking the teacher. The scene was frozen there at the cliffhanger.

The students were hooked. "This is our scene work. Are you interested?" Carlos said. Most students nodded in agreement, and we invited them to join the circle. A few students remained at their desks, including a small-framed student wearing a red hoodie pulled down over his face.

Jose was watching intently from an open spot under his hoodie. Carlos, in an effort to empower him, asked him if he might want to participate as the director of the next scene. Jose reluctantly agreed and said, "Quiet on the set, action!" as instructed.

Two students replayed the scene, and the class processed potential solutions to the conflict. As the process moved forward, Jose became fully engaged.

Next, we asked the class what other issues they wanted to address.

"Parents!" Jose pushed back his hood and yelled out from his seat. "My mother never listens to me and always screams at me, telling me I'm no good. She is just like the teacher in the scene."

We took the cue and constructed an on-the-spot scene about a son wanting to attend a neighborhood party. Jose was invited to play the son, with Carlos standing behind him as his coach. The scene opens with the son on his way out to go to a party when, at the last minute, his mom tells him that she needs him to stay home and watch his little brother again. When he pushes back, she threatens to tell his father, who the son appears to be very afraid of, based on his frozen response. At that point, the scene turns unexpectedly away from the usual ENACT formula. Jose starts to run out of the house, and his mother calls after him, but he suddenly stops. There is silence; we see Jose standing there. Carlos tries to help him explain his feelings to the mom, but Jose collapses on the floor.

The room is silent. Jose is lying on the floor. We all look at him, including the teacher, and wonder what is happening. Is he OK?

After a few moments, he gets up, crawling on his knees, frantically looking for something on the ground. "I can't find them. I can't find my LEGS!"

I play along. "Oh no!" I responded. "Can we help you find them?"

Several students jump from their seats and search for Jose's lost legs. We are all crawling around the floor, looking for his imaginary legs, when he suddenly stands up and announces, "I found them! I found my legs!"

We all clap, despite having no idea what is going on. Jose jumps up proudly and runs out the door, repeating, "I found them, I found them!" The bell rings as if on cue, and the class ends. Jose found his legs that day with the help of his classmates, but what he really found was his power!

We never found out if Jose was in a gang, but we hoped that discovering his power through a metaphor of finding his legs with the support of his peers might have given him a new, more positive self-concept that he was profoundly lacking. The school counselor let us know that she would follow up with him.

Author's Notes

- Chaotic classroom behavior can become a pattern. Sometimes, just the proper interruption can break the pattern. The actor's surprise entrance broke the pattern with an engaging scene.
- The scene took an unexpected turn when a withdrawn student unwittingly worked through his issue of powerlessness by losing and finding his legs.
- Sometimes, going with the group's flow and letting go of a formulated process is needed.
- Trauma lives in the body and, if left unaddressed, can cause unmanageable symptoms. Jose revealed his trauma by demonstrating an unconscious trauma response, the collapse response, by falling onto the floor.
- We suspected Jose of being in a gang and hoped that with the support of his classmates, he would feel the sense of attachment and belonging he craved. This new sense of belonging might help him feel less inclined to need the support of a gang.

Aisha: The Motherless Child

Underlying Need: Connection

"This kid is driving me nuts; she will not stop following me around; she is like a stalker," the principal, Ms. Miller, told me. Aisha stood apart from the other youth in a group of students described as "highly acting out." Ms. Miller described them as "a volcano group on the verge of exploding."

Aisha was quiet and attentive and had remarkable artistic talent, as I discovered the first day when I glimpsed at some of her sketches. When I asked Ms. Miller why Aisha was part of the "volcano" group, she said, "Be careful. Aisha is a compulsive liar." I wondered what she meant.

Aisha had told everyone in school that Ms. Miller was her special aunt. She even announced over the loudspeaker that she was Ms. Miller's favorite niece. Her lies began when she was moved into a new foster home a year before. (She had been forced to move to several foster homes.) She had been calling the principal day and night and hanging up. "I want her behavior to stop! She is stalking me," Ms. Miller had told me.

The distressed principal pulled a lovely portrait of herself from her desk and showed it to me. "Here, look at this; she drew this of me. She won't leave me alone!" A crumpled piece of paper portrayed a kind-faced, wide-eyed woman with long black hair. "This was done from memory." The well-executed portrait of Ms. Miller did not help the principal empathize.

I stared at the portrait and wondered what it must be like to have no mother figure to come home to. Aisha had been moved four or five times to different foster families. She didn't know where her birth mother was. Aisha wasn't on the same playing field as other kids who benefited from positive early childhood experiences with their caretakers. She lived with a constant fear of abandonment.

Aisha desperately needed an intimate connection with another human being to affirm her existence. She craved to be seen, heard, and validated. Sadly, the principal must not have understood this, or been aware of attachment theory, which explains the devastating effects that a lack of early childhood bonding can have. We now have a much better understanding of the effects of childhood attachment insecurity and exposure to trauma in early childhood, which interferes with the ability to form secure attachments.

Ms. Miller dashed off to an emergency. My partner and I went to the "volcano classroom" and began our work there, which would take place over a few weeks. Aisha and I developed a relationship primarily through discussing her artwork. Each day, I would ask what she was working on, and she was excited to show me. One day, she opened up to me and said she wanted to attend a high school where she could focus on her art. I concurred that it was a great idea, and I arranged a meeting with the guidance counselor to discuss this with her the following week. But the day that Aisha was supposed to meet with the counselor, Aisha was not in class. She was nowhere to be found. When I asked Ms. Miller about Aisha, she told me Aisha had switched from stalking her to stalking the gym teacher, a woman who yelled at her, pushing her away. Aisha had had a panic attack, fainted, and was taken to the emergency room.

The group work continued for the last week without Aisha. I never saw her again, but I always remembered her. I thought about how, if she had returned, we could have tried to help her feel connected to the group, that she belonged somewhere. I imagined scenarios where she would draw pictures of our workshops and visualized her holding up her drawing while the group applauded. I wanted to see her feel appreciated and take a bow. But it never happened. I got caught up in the swirls of the work and had to admit some sense of defeat as Aisha faded into another story of working with youth with trauma.

Author's Notes

Because Aisha was moved from one foster home to another starting as a child, she suffered from attachment trauma. Readers will recognize from this story the degree to which youth fool others or themselves as a form of protection from emotional pain that, unfortunately, is self-destructive. They often lack the necessary emotional awareness and vocabulary to express themselves. These are cases in which they need extra help, empathy, and compassion from adults.

- Aisha suffered from a lack of attachment that started as a child and followed her into her youth, moving from foster home to foster home. She felt like a "motherless child" and needed to feel loved and cared about. She desperately searched for someone to play this role.

- The principal did not understand the devastating effects of attachment trauma. By telling Aisha to stop her inexplicably needy behavior, she was rubbing salt in Aisha's attachment wounds by pushing her away and alienating her further.
- Understanding Aisha's needs and *attuning to* her would have helped Aisha enormously, but the principal was overwhelmed. She did not have the emotional bandwidth or the tools to help her.
- Often, the children who "act out," like Aisha, are missing something basic from their lives, like the safety, trust, connection, and empathy that stem from early childhood/caregiver connection.
- Aisha had a "collapse response," a trauma response that is considered "the defense response of last resort," when she fainted after trying everything to connect to someone else who thwarted her once again.

Stewart: The Rocket Boy

Underlying Need: Safety

Although some children suffer from symptoms caused by attention-deficit hyperactivity disorder (ADHD), upon further investigation, many children are overwhelmed with internal feelings that cause dysregulated behavior. Enter Stewart, an elementary school student in the South Bronx.

In the early 1990s, as ADHD became a standard label, I mainly worked with special education students diagnosed with learning or behavioral disabilities. With a few years' experience behind me, I generally could read a group within minutes to register their emotional state.

Along with Roger, my teaching-artist partner, I was hired by the school principal to teach life skills to a high-energy group of 10-year-olds at a South Bronx elementary school. Knowing our audience, we started a simple unison clapping game to create a safe container with explicit physical boundaries. We laid down some basic rules for them, like no pushing or hitting. These rules usually worked with kids of this age group. But one skinny boy with tousled hair kept darting out of the circle, saying, "I'm Rocket Boy." His teacher would grab him and mutter, "Stewart, be still!" It happened once every two minutes, and Stewart's outbursts seemed to exacerbate the rest of the group's easy distractibility. The teacher pulled Stewart onto her lap to contain him.

I pivoted to a different game: the energy ball exercise, designed for just this sort of antsy group. The kids followed my request to shake their hands and get ready to catch an imaginary energy ball. "Whatever part of the body the energy ball touches will get shaken up," I explained. They shook the "ball" on their hands, heads, and legs, laughing as the imaginary ball was passed around the circle.

But Stewart, trapped in his teacher's lap, could not sit still and could not participate. We could either continue to thwart his pent-up energy or find a way to release it naturally, but which would be more effective?

Before choosing, I wanted to assess if Stewart was aware of his excessively active internal state. We asked the kids to sit on the floor in a circle, and Roger and I did a theatrical experiment. Roger created a metaphor for feeling uncontained by playing the character of an out-of-control machine. I explained that it was a special machine with a little problem. It could not stop moving, and I asked them if they could help him. They agreed. All together, we yelled out, "One, two, three, action!" Unable to contain himself, Stewart jumped out of his teacher's lap to join us.

"I like to move," said Roger the machine. As he moved around the room in all directions, the students giggled. Then he began to move faster and faster. "Sometimes I need to move very fast, very, very fast, but then I can't slow down. My engine won't stop!" The kids watched in fascination. Then, the machine began to speed up, jumping and hopping around the room. "Oh no," he said. "I can't stop. I don't know how."

"What's going on?" I asked the children.

"He can't stop moving," a student said. "Why not?" "He has too much energy," said another student. I asked what that felt like. "Nervous," a child responded. "Do you ever feel this way?" Several of them raised their hands. "What should we do to help Roger the machine slow down?"

"Tell him to stop!" they yelled.

"I have a stop word," I said. "Freeze!" I called out.

Roger stopped. But after a few moments, Roger started to move again. I yelled "Freeze!" a second time, and he stopped again. "Why don't you help me?" I asked the children. "Can you say 'freeze' with me?"

We all yelled "Freeze!" together. Roger froze again. "Why don't we try it? Let's all jump as fast as we can, and when I say freeze, you all freeze. Ok, everybody jump, faster, faster!" They jumped, I yelled, "Freeze!" and they all froze, including Stewart.

Then, I gave them a tool to use themselves. I told them they had an imaginary button on their shoulder that they could tap to slow down. "When you think you can't stop moving like Roger, tap the control button, and it will help you stop. Let's try it. Ok, here goes. One, two, three, move!"

The children moved quickly around the room. "Faster," I directed. They moved faster. "Ok, hit the button!" They hit their buttons, stopped moving immediately, and then fell to the floor laughing.

Roger took the cue of them lying on the floor and suggested the children stay there and close their eyes. We had other options: They could sit in their chairs if that felt more comfortable and keep their eyes open if that made them feel safer. Roger guided them through a peaceful meditation, taking them through imaginary lush grass fields where they heard running water from a nearby stream. They were guided to feel safe and relaxed.

All the students lay still, and their otherwise jittery hands and legs rested. Except for Stewart, who seemed to feel afraid the moment he relaxed. He shot up from the floor.

"I don't like to close my eyes; it makes me feel scared," he said.

Stewart couldn't stop moving because he felt unsafe inside. Perhaps he never learned to self-regulate or find inner safety because of negative early attachment. Perhaps something traumatic happened to him.

"It's ok," I said. I'm here with you." I sat beside him with my hand on his shoulder, breathing slowly and evenly with him until he relaxed. The bell rang.

I never learned Stewart's history, but I knew something kept him on hyperalert. The bell rang, and the kids got up and ran to lunch.

Following the session, I spoke with Stewart's teacher, who had been intently observing the session and noted the change she saw in the students' behavior. I suggested she continue using some of our games and offered her other techniques she could use to help them all feel safe. She learned a new perspective about hyperactivity: It may be more than what meets the eye, and further investigation is necessary before making a conclusive diagnosis.

On our last day working with this group of children, I suggested she consult with the school counselor and devise a plan to ensure Stewart's safety in and out of school. She made sure to follow up with the school counselor right away.

Author's Notes

- The ENACT Method uses symbols and metaphors when working with children because it is a non-literal language they understand.
- Though a child may be diagnosed with ADHD or hyperactivity, adults should not ignore other issues, such as developmental trauma, that may be the root cause of their symptoms.
- When Stewart said he was scared to close his eyes and relax, it may have been a clue pointing to early trauma.
- An imaginary tool, a "control button," was used to help students develop self-efficacy and learn to self-regulate.

- Safety measures should be enforced during all activities with children. There are various ways to help them feel safe when participating. In the guided visual meditation mentioned in this chapter, students were invited to sit on the floor or in their chairs and keep their eyes open or shut, depending on their comfort level.
- If you suspect abuse, report it immediately to the appropriate personnel in the school or institution.

Marcus: The Superhero
Underlying Need: Connection

"He's a talented artist," my colleague Jenna had mentioned about Marcus, the tall, large-boned Latinx teenager who sat huddled on the floor, his head buried in a sketchbook. I also knew that Marcus, like the other students in this group, had severe emotional problems. He was put in a hospital program because he would barely speak to anyone unless he pretended to be a superhero robot character he had created and had depicted obsessively in cartoon sketches.

Jenna, my other two colleagues, and I worked with Marcus to help him overcome his resistance to socially interacting with others. We had agreed with the students to work together to create a small theater production that we would put on for one another as well as for some invited friends and family. Marcus was an amiable, smiling, and shy boy who stayed withdrawn throughout most initial games. "Yes," "No," "Guess so," "I draw," and "I'm Robot Man" were about the extent of his responses to any questions. Except for his occasional smile, his body and body language seemed rigid and constricted. He moved like a machine and spoke in a monotone. He had worked hard to create a superhero role, presenting as someone who was impervious to harm.

Each day, I asked to see his sketches. A vibrant, orange-yellow figure with hard, squared arms, torso, and head fended off weaselly-looking bad guys. "What's going on here?" I would ask. "Robot Man-has-a-lot-of-strength. He-uses-it-for-good." Marcus's voice was Robot Man's, and he lifted his head long enough for me to see a slight shine in his eyes. Robot Man's body, I realized, was also hard and rigid, and yet his spirit pulsated from within. Once we invited Marcus to introduce himself each day as Robot Man, he gradually participated more and more.

He would play some theater games as Robot Man but always remained detached from himself and the group. It was as if he were going through the motions but not really present. The group accepted him nonetheless.

But the real breakthrough came in a drawing that involved Robot Man's family and the follow-up to the scene. The sketch depicted a family of robots standing rigidly together in a family photo. He had also created roles for his parents. Taking our cue from his sketch, my team recreated his Robot family.

Ellen and Henry were extremely compassionate teaching artists who trusted each other and their intuition to create a scene on the spot to connect with Marcus. Ellen embodied the role of Robot Man's mother, and Henry played his Robot father. Intuitively, without planning, they knew exactly what to do. They would prepare Marcus, Robot Man, for school.

Ellen and Harry sensed that Marcus needed nurturing. Portraying rigid-bodied robot parents, Harry, Robot Man's father, gently placed his son's backpack on his shoulders. With a monotone voice and robot-like gestures, Ellen, Robot Man's mom, brushed his hair and packed his school lunchbox. Each food item was warm and hearty, "Just what a growing robot son needs," she said. Then, Robot Man's father gently placed each book, one by one, in Robot Man's backpack, adding pens, pencils, and drawing paper to the mix. They got him ready to take him to the school bus. Robot Man appeared happy. As the imaginary bus arrived, Robot Man's mom and dad kissed him on the cheek and waved a long goodbye, wishing him a good day. He waved back.

After the scene with the three performers concluded, I asked the superhero family if they could unzip their imaginary robot costumes, knowing that they could still maintain their superhero qualities of strength and radiance. "You can slip the costume back on whenever you like," I told them. Robot Man's mom helped him unzip his costume. They each unzipped their own and introduced themselves by their real names. Ellen looked at Marcus and asked, "Do you have another name? Could you tell us? "Marcus, my name is Marcus," he said in a deeper, authentic-sounding voice.

Of course, Robot Man's family life might have shone compared to Marcus's. A few weeks later, Marcus's father showed up early to watch the play. His dark eyes, sparse hair, dried skin, emaciated frame, and constricted breathing signaled he was not well. "I have AIDS. I might not have long. I want to see the performance," he said, combing his thinning hair to look presentable among the other parents and students. I showed him the large sketches Marcus had made as a theatrical backdrop for our performance. His father, for a moment, lit up and smiled. He was proud.

Like all of us, Marcus had his demons he wanted to fight away—the demons of illness, suffering, alienation, and death. He wanted to shine and be strong in ways his father could no longer be. He deeply desired to be a superhero. That evening, Marcus brought his father joy and a moment of relief during his last days, and his father saw and understood a side of his son he likely had never witnessed before.

Author's Notes

Marcus's story epitomizes what happens when trauma causes youth to retreat into a deep fantasy world of their own making. These fantasy worlds are usually delicately constructed. Trying to wrench a youth from a fantasy further alienates them. So, parents, teachers, and counselors must strike a balance between not completely indulging a youth in the fantasy, not trying to destroy the fantasy world, and not simply ignoring the fantasy.

In the story, you saw how we:

- Gently engaged Marcus's role and honored his fantasy world.
- Acknowledged his creative talent—art, imagination, problem-solving, music, story-telling—involved in his world creation.
- Identified the positive qualities of the created role.
- Encouraged Marcus to realize that assuming the alternative persona can be a choice and that he could embody the same powerful qualities as the persona he created.
- The story shows readers the next step: Helping youth see that persona is an acceptable choice when needed, but a choice nonetheless. They can choose not to be stuck in the role.

Group Case History: Transforming Collective Trauma

In addition to experiencing individual trauma, a youth may have experienced a traumatic event that affects an entire community, such as a school or neighborhood.

My experiences working in schools in the aftermath of collective trauma led me to see how an extreme event leads to extreme behavior in students as a group. One example was the case history of the teens affected by the attacks on the World Trade Center, included in an earlier chapter. In this case, as in others, the students shut down, resonating with each other's fears and somehow understanding each other's defenses. They remain silent, disassociating or retreating as a shield against untenable feelings, which, if they emerge, can break open the floodgates, causing them to re-experience the trauma.

But extreme events called for extreme strength and resilience. I felt honored for the opportunity to work with individuals who were able to overcome what seemed to be insurmountable obstacles. Their bravery, humor, talent, and sense of fun created group solidarity that led us, in some cases, to create community theater together. In many cases, these theater pieces addressed issues of social justice. Sharing common experiences, both challenging and hopeful, led to collective healing. What follows is another of these stories.

The Confused Ones[1]

Underlying Need: Protection

"The parents are coming into school with baseball bats!" the principal of a Bronx school exclaimed. "A kid was shot in our school parking lot yesterday, and parents are showing up ready to take action right now!"

My teaching partner Charles and I arrived at a high school in the South Bronx for our first day of work. The principal, Ms. Emory, told us that the parents were furious about the incident and wanted retaliation. They told their kids to carry baseball bats to school, but the school administration wouldn't allow them to enter the building if they had them. "The kids are confused. They are either not talking, going home sick, or not showing up to school at all," Ms. Emory exclaimed.

When we entered the room, the students were silent. They sat at their desks, drawing and writing notes, and some had their heads down on their desks. Some students were sleeping. Several students complained to the teacher that their stomachs hurt and they needed to go to the nurse's office. This was a group in distress. We needed to help them move out of their current condition. We would engage them in a scene.

We started with our tried-and-true conflict scene between a teacher and a disruptive student. My partner Charles jumped immediately into the scene and enlisted me as the frustrated teacher, trying to get his attention. He played a loud, boisterous, clown-like student. Charles used his comedy to demonstrate the clown-like defense around his character's inner feelings of distress. Ignoring the teacher, he danced around the room with headphones on, cracking jokes and sitting beside other students.

We could see that the class was engaged entirely in the ENACT process as they described the character's behavior and inner feelings. They worked to solve the conflict between the student and the teacher, replaying the scene with various solutions.

Now we needed to move on to the critical goal of unpacking the current situation unfolding in the school and neighborhood. We had to construct a scene, identify the core feelings that were causing them to shut down, and help students become aware of their defenses to address their underlying feelings and make sense of them.

Students were getting contradictory messages from their parents and their teachers. Parents told them to bring baseball bats to school for protection, and teachers warned them they would be in serious trouble if they did.

The mixed messaging led to the feeling of **cognitive dissonance**. Without knowing who to answer to or how to make sense of their feelings, they were coping with enormous stress, and most of the students shut down or somaticized the feelings by experiencing physical symptoms. We needed to develop a theatrical medicine to help students understand and express their emotions to relieve their confusion and distress.

Upon our return the following week for the next session, the principal reported that several students were still not attending school, and many were shut down emotionally. Students continued to be in and out of the nurse's office, complaining of stomach aches and other physical ailments. The nurse was overwhelmed; teachers did not know what to do. They needed support. We knew it was unlikely that any change in behavior would occur unless we unearthed the core feeling of cognitive dissonance.

The incident created overwhelming collective trauma; we needed to be mindful of using enough distance in the scene to help the class connect without feeling overwhelmed. Changing all the critical elements of the situation, we designed the scene to occur in the retail store where Johanna, a high school student, has just gotten her first job and is happy. Her parents are proud of her, and she plans to use the money for college.

Suddenly, her close friend Charisse enters the store and begins eyeing the merchandise. She tells Johanna to look the other way as she steals a sweater off the rack. She explains she needs to wear a new sweater to a party. Johanna is shocked by her request and turns her down. Charisse retaliates.

Charisse threatens Johanna that if she does not let her take the sweater, she will end their friendship and tell all her friends that Johanna betrayed her and can't be trusted as a friend. Johanna tries to explain that she wants to give Charisse the sweater, but it could cost her job and could even get her in trouble with the police. Charisse continues the pressure, and Johanna doesn't know what to do. She sees her manager looking at her sternly from the back of the store. The scene is frozen, and an inner monologue exposes Johanna's core feeling and its connection to her physical symptoms.

I know she needs this sweater for the party. It is important to her cuz everyone will be there. She is my best friend. I don't want to lose her. I don't know what to do. I need this job. If my boss finds out, he will fire me immediately and report me to the police. When my parents find out, I'll be grounded. They will be so disappointed with me. I don't know what to do. I want to give her the sweater; she will start rumors about me if I don't. I feel sick. My stomach hurts, and my head is beginning to pound. I don't know what to do.

In the scene processing, we discussed feelings of confusion and indecision. I asked the students if they had ever experienced anything like this.

"A kid was killed in our school parking lot last week," one student said. "All the parents in the neighborhood are upset. One parent told the other parents to tell us kids to come to school with baseball bats to protect ourselves. The principal said we were not allowed." Another student said, "We are all upset. We don't know what to do and don't want to come to school. A lot of us feel sick."

We knew it could be helpful if the students could see the connection between their physical symptoms and their emotions. We hoped that helping students identify their core feelings and talking about the experience would relieve them from their symptoms and give them the chance to have a voice—the first step toward any kind of action. Of course, there was still a more significant situation of fear, anger and violence playing out in the school and the community that needed to be addressed if real change was to occur. We couldn't do more alone.

Collective trauma can be especially challenging to address when it brings up conscious or unconscious memories of prior traumas, as was the case in this situation. For example, historical trauma based on issues of inequality and racism may have been lurking in the unconscious. In order to heal, the next step would be for the school and community to work together to address the issues that led to the incident. These could include issues such as being under-resourced and police violence.

Author's Notes

- To address trauma, it is essential to understand the core emotion that underlies the behavior.
- Cognitive dissonance was the unexpressed emotion causing the students to shut down. Unable to deal with their emotions, they somatized their feelings and had physical symptoms.
- Using the ENACT role-play method helped unearth the core emotions underneath the trauma symptoms.
- Collective trauma takes a community to promote change. The ENACT Method helped students identify their feelings of confusion and get out of their "frozen" state, and now the school and community needed to take the necessary steps toward change.

Note

1 Feldman, *Current Approaches in Drama Therapy*, 293.

Appendix 3

Sample Lesson Plans

Lesson Plan 1. Facing Fears

Addressing the Defense of AVOIDANCE

The Goal

Youth will understand how the *avoidance defense* prevents them from connecting.

Skill

Youth will learn to *name and communicate their feelings.*

Warm-Up

Choose from the list of games in Appendix 1—specifically browsing three choices in Chapter 7, *Defenses.*

The Scene

A student is called on by their classroom teacher to read their poem in front of the class. They are afraid that their peers will laugh and mock them, and they resist getting up. The student displays various avoidant behaviors. They shuffle through their papers, drop their notebook on the floor, and ask to go to the bathroom. The teacher becomes frustrated and yells at the student to hurry up. After the teacher's second and third requests, the student freezes. The scene stops, and the student does an inner monologue.

Inner Monologue

I can't read my poem in front of the class. It's personal, and the kids will all laugh at it. I want to do it, but I know I am going to be made fun of. My hands are shaking, and I am starting to feel sick. I've got to get out of here!

The scene is unfrozen, and the student yells at the teacher. "Leave me alone!"

Processing

The facilitator plays a vital role at this stage, guiding participants to identify the core feelings of fear and shame and to name the avoidant behaviors that covered up those feelings (shuffling through papers, asking to go to the nurses' office, etc.). Once the group understands the core feeling of shame and the avoidant defense, they are guided toward solutions for managing fear and shame. The facilitator guides them in a replay, naming the core feelings and telling the teacher how they felt.

The scene is replayed a few times, with various students telling the teacher how they feel.

Closure

Recommended: Have students go around the circle and name one thing they do if they feel nervous.

Lesson Plan 2. It's Your Fault!

Addressing the Defense of BLAME

The Goal

Students will understand the *blame defense*.

Skill

To learn to *take accountability* for feelings.

Warm-Up

Choose from the available theater games.

The Scene

Two students are in art class and have to work together to paint a picture which would be hung in the school hallway. They have differing views over who did the art and whether they should use more colors. They push and pull, and after a while, the paper ripped into pieces. The students blame each other, and the teacher asks who ripped it. One of the girls blames the other. "She did it; it was her fault." They continue to yell and almost get into a fistfight. The scene is frozen.

This scene does not need an inner monologue.

Processing

The facilitator processes the scene, focusing on the blame defense and asking why people blame each other. The goal is for them to learn to take accountability for their feelings and actions. They are asked to replay the scene, with each student apologizing and taking ownership of their feelings.

Closure

Students go around the circle and say: "One thing I learned today was...."

Lesson Plan 3. Cutting Class
Addressing the Defense of INDIFFERENCE

The Goal

Students will understand the defense of *indifference*.

Skill

Students will learn to *name and communicate their feelings*.

Warm-Up

Attitude sculptures.

The Scene

A student has been asked to meet with the dean to address why they have been cutting classes.

The student makes up various excuses for missing class. The dean responds that cutting classes is unacceptable and warns the student that any future instances will result in strong consequences, including suspension. The dean explains that they won't get into college if they miss school. The student responds with apathy, saying, "I don't care!" The scene is frozen, and the student does an inner monologue.

Inner Monologue

Why is this dean picking on me? He doesn't like me, I can tell! I'm so behind in class that I'll fail the test again, so why should I bother? No one can help me at home; my mom doesn't speak English. I'll never get into college, so why bother?

The scene ends with the student walking out of the dean's office, shaking his head.

Processing

Facilitators guide participants in naming the behavior and the core feeling of hopelessness expressed by the student in the inner monologue. After students are asked if and how they relate to the scene, they are invited to do a replay communicating the character's feelings to the dean.

Closure

Magic Box.

Lesson Plan 4. The Show

Addressing Symptoms of HYPERAROUSAL

The Goal

Students will *identify symptoms of hyperarousal.*

Skills

Students will learn skills to *manage anxiety.*

Warm-Up

Students are asked to "cross the line" if they have ever experienced feelings of stress, such as anxiety.

The Scene

Two friends, Sheila and Eve, are about to go onstage for the neighborhood talent show. They are about to do a dance they made up, which they have practiced for months. Backstage, Sheila is excited and practicing their moves. Eve is becoming increasingly nervous and is pacing back and forth nonstop, jabbering. Her breathing becomes faster, her heart is racing. "Are you okay?" Sheila asks. "Come on, you got this!" Eve replies that she is not ready and then breaks into an inner monologue expressing her anxiety.

Inner Monologue

I can't do this; I feel sick! My palms are all sweaty, I'm nauseous, and my heart is racing! I feel like I'm going to pass out. I don't want to let my friends down; it means so much to them, and we have been working so hard, but I'm so frightened and afraid I'm going to black out!

Sheila says, "Come on, Eve, we are in this together." Eve replies, "I think I am going to faint." Sheila takes her hands and asks if they can breathe together. We see Eve calm down.

The scene ends with Sheila saying, "I got your back; if you need to get off the stage, I'll do it myself, but at least try." Eve agrees.

Processing

The facilitator guides the participants in exploring various symptoms of anxiety, including those identified in the monologue. The symptoms can be written on the blackboard or flip chart. Then, the group is asked to explore various coping strategies, including taking deep breaths, self-talk, counting to 10, etc. These are also written on the board. The facilitator asks the group if they can remember a time they have felt anxiety, but instead of sharing out loud, they are asked to write it on a piece of paper and then choose a coping strategy they could use if it ever happens again. The facilitator invites students up to replay the scene, focusing on deep breaths as a skill to calm down.

Closure

A grounding meditation.

Lesson Plan 5. My Way or the Highway

Recognizing Signs of RELATIONSHIP ABUSE

The Goal

Participants will recognize signs of *relationship abuse.*

Skills

Participants will learn to *walk away if they feel unsafe* and *report the perpetrator if necessary.*

Warm-Up

"Yes/No" game.

The Scene

A young man is on the phone with his girlfriend. He does not want his girlfriend to hang out with her friends or do anything alone without him. He says it is because he "loves her" and always wants to be with her. When she pushes back, saying she wants to be with her friends without him and needs some time alone, he becomes increasingly angry, threatening that he will tell all her friends what a "child" she is. When he doesn't get her agreement, he threatens to hurt her if he sees her alone. The scene ends where she stands frozen.

This scene does not require an inner monologue.

Processing

The facilitator guides the participants to recognize where abuse occurred in the scene and how the boyfriend tried to manipulate his girlfriend. They are asked to give other examples of relationship abuse before coming up with strategies to stop it. This scene can have a reply with the girlfriend standing up for herself and then walking away, but it is not required.

IMPORTANT: The facilitator should let the group know that if they or anyone they know are dealing with any abuse, it should be reported immediately to the National Domestic Violence Hotline: 800-799-7233.

Closure

Hand squeeze.

Additional Resources

Trauma Resources

- National Child Traumatic Stress Network (NCTSN). Treatment for youth, training, and education. http://www.nctsnet.org/
- American Psychological Association. Resources guides. http://www.nctsnet.org
- ACE Study http://acestoohigh.com/got-your-ace-score/; http://www.cdc.gov/violenceprevention/acestudy
- HelpPRO therapist finder. Local therapists specializing in trauma, serving specific age groups, http://www.helppro.com/
- National Institute of Mental Health: http://www.nimh.nih.gov/health/topics/post-traumatic-stress-disorder-ptsd/index.shtml

Somatic Approaches to Trauma

- Sensorimotor Institute: Pat Ogden, creator of the Sensorimotor Psychotherapy method. A therapeutic modality for trauma, providing training in Sensorimotor Psychotherapy drawing from somatic therapies and other therapeutic approaches. www.sensorimotorpsychotherapy.org/about
- Somatic Experiencing: A somatic approach to healing trauma developed by Peter Levine. https://traumahealing.org

Drama Therapy

- National Association of Drama Therapy. https://www.nadta.org
- World Alliance of Drama Therapy. https://worldallianceofdramatherapy.com

Expressive Arts Therapy

- Trauma-Informed Practices and Expressive Arts Therapy Institute: Developed by Cathy Malchiodi: Trauma-informed practices, "brain-wise" and arts-based intervention training. www.trauma-informed-practice.com

Teaching Artist Associations

- ITAC collaborative: ITAC's mission is to support, expand, and connect the international community of teaching artists. https://itac-collaborative.com
- The New York City Arts in Education Roundtable: To elevate, enhance, and sustain the work of the arts education community in New York City's schools and communities. https://www.nycaieroundtable.org

Improvisation Classes

- The Second City New York, based in various cities. Offers classes and shows. https://www.secondcity.com
- The Upright Citizens Brigade. Offers all levels of improvisation. ucbcomedy.com
- Magnet Theater. https://magnettheater.com/class/improv-level-one/?gad_source=1&gbraid=0AAAAADwLS08AEv24pVjPEeR_U3a1cmFpx

Index

Note: Page numbers followed by "n" refer to notes.